Xandria Williams began her career as a geochemist involved in mineral exploration but then turned to biochemistry and the study of human nutrition and health, followed by naturopathy, homoeopathy and botanic medicine. She then extended her studies to neurolinguistic programming, voice dialogue and many other methods of helping people with emotional, personal and psychological as well as physical health problems.

She has lectured extensively at many natural therapies colleges and conferences and holds classes and seminars on a range of aspects of physical, mental and emotional health care.

She has written over three hundred and fifty articles, has often been heard on radio and television and is the author of *Living with Allergies, What's in My Food, Choosing Health Intentionally, Choosing Weight Intentionally, Stress: Recognise and Resolve, Love, Health and Happiness, Beating the Blues, Fatigue, Eating Right* and *You're Not Alone.*

Xandria Williams has evolved her unique and highly effective approach to tackling life's problems during twenty-five years of research into helping people at her clinics in Sydney and London. She has drawn extensively on this background while writing this book and has brought together the many and different solutions that have evolved during her years of experience in helping people to solve the daily challenges of dealing with candida.

Xandria is now in practice in central London and can be contacted for consultations or for copies of her books on tel/fax (00 44) 0171 824 8153.

OVERCOMING CANDIDA

THE ULTIMATE COOKERY GUIDE

Xandria Williams

ELEMENT

Shaftesbury, Dorset • Boston, Massachusetts
Melbourne, Victoria

© Element Books Limited 1998
Text © Xandria Williams 1998

First published in Great Britain in 1998 by
Element Books Limited
Shaftesbury, Dorset SP7 8BP

Published in the USA in 1998 by
Element Books, Inc.
160 North Washington Street, Boston MA 02114

Published in Australia in 1998 by
Element Books
and distributed by Penguin Australia Limited
487 Maroondah Highway, Ringwood, Victoria 3134

Cover design by Slatter-Anderson
Text illustrations by Lucinda Bothwell
Design by Roger Lightfoot
Typeset by Footnote Graphics, Warminster, Wilts
Printed and bound in Great Britain by
Creative Print and Design (Wales), Ebbw Vale

British Library Cataloguing in Publication
data available

Library of Congress Cataloging in Publication
data available

ISBN 1-86204-172-5

Contents

Foreword

'Well, Geraldine,' I said to the woman facing me across the desk, 'you are not "going mad" as you feared; nor have you become a "thoroughly nasty person", as you tell me your husband has claimed from time to time. Equally, your problem is not "all in your mind", as your doctor told you. From what you have told me and the tests we have done, it seems that your major problem is candidiasis.'

'What's that?' Geraldine looked confused and uncertain.

I explained that it was a condition caused by a normally harmless mould or yeast, of which *Candida albicans* was the most common and troublesome, that had colonized her digestive tract and become a dominant species. I also explained the consequences, including the physiological and chemical reactions that resulted in her mood swings and in the failing memory and mental confusion that had led her to doubt her own sanity. Finally I reassured her that the uncomfortable and embarrassing digestive and bowel problems she was having were not, as she had begun to fear, some dreadful and sinister disease, but were also the result of the candidiasis.

'What do I do now? Is there something I should take?'

'There are certainly some things you should take,' I said, and gave her a list of them, together with details of where to get them and how to take them. 'There are also a number of things you should do, and these include, I'm sorry to have to tell you, some major dietary restrictions and changes.'

By the time I had finished detailing these I could see her looking distressed.

'But what *can* I eat?' she wailed.

I gave her the list of foods she couldn't eat, a list of foods she could eat, and several pages of suggestions and recipes that had been compiled during the past twenty years and in the process of helping hundreds of people. Seeing some sort of help and support was at hand she began to look more hopeful and once again, as many times before, I promised myself that one day I would put all the ideas together into a book. Soon after that the opportunity arose, and this book is the result.

A Note on Measurements

This book uses metric, Imperial, and American measurements. Dry ingredients are measured in grams/ounces, grams/ounces/ US cups, or Imperial spoons/US spoons; Imperial spoons are rounded or heaped and US spoons level. Liquid ingredients are measured either in millilitres/Imperial fluid ounces/US fluid ounces or millilitres/Imperial fluid ounces/US cups (1 Imperial pint = 20 fluid ounces = 0.568 litre; 1 US pint = 16 fluid ounces = 0.550 litre), or millilitres/Imperial spoons/US cups or millilitres/Imperial spoons/US spoons.

A Note on Measurements

How This Book Will Help

Candidiasis was recognized over two thousand years ago by the Greek physician Hippocrates, who described 'thrush' in the mouth and the vagina; but it has never been so common as in recent decades. Our modern diet is the reason: a lower consumption of essential nutrients and a higher consumption of sugar, sugar-rich foods and refined carbohydrates (including white flour), and a reliance on high-yeast or yeast-encouraging foods such as bread, cheese, smoked meat and fish, dried fruit and a variety of yeast-based and fermented sauces available in ready-to-use form in bottles on the shop shelves. Digestive incompetence, including inadequate production of stomach acid, poor digestion and pandemic constipation, high levels of stress, and the contraceptive pill and antibiotics are the other main causes.

Many people suffering from candidiasis do not receive a proper diagnosis and this can result in years of unnecessary ill health and distress. Others start on the treatment, somewhat overwhelmed by the changes they must make, but with every intention of continuing; however without support and guidance on the lifestyle changes involved, on a near daily basis, they frequently give up.

Around twenty years ago, when I first started dealing with the problem of candidiasis in my practice, there were no practical books available to recommend to patients. There were very few of the special foods I recommend in *Overcoming Candida*, which are now widely available, such as alternatives to the forbidden cow's milk products. There were certainly no recipe books, and it took hours to get a patient set up with recipes and with food alternatives, so I began to put together a variety of printed sheets with recipes and meal suggestions. The list grew, until eventually it was time to put these ideas into a book.

Nearly all the suggestions here, and many of the recipes, have developed out of a common need: mine, as the practitioner faced with the patients' questions, and my patients', who had been told what the problem was, and were armed with a list of what to avoid, but had no guide to what to eat instead. Now I have put all this information together and given it to you, your life, though possibly complicated by all you have to do, will be a lot simpler than it might otherwise be. As well as guiding you through the effective treatments, this book will show you how to shop, cook, eat out, snack, socialize and handle all the possible problems associated with a candida diet. This book, I hope, will fill the gap.

PART ONE

What is Candida?

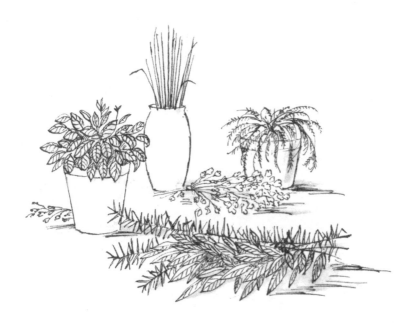

CHAPTER 1

Something is Wrong

When you go to a doctor with a specific pain, problem or group of symptoms you will usually come away with a name for the disease or condition that is causing the symptoms and either a prescription for a medication or a referral for tests or to a specialist. The story is very different if you have a wide range of symptoms, particularly if none is dominant or even especially strong, if they don't affect a specific organ or part of the body and if they don't fit into the expected pattern of one of the medically recognized and named diseases. Even though they're causing you concern, even though they're pulling you down and leaving you feeling unwell, you may find yourself going from one practitioner to another and yet not getting a satisfactory diagnosis, treatment or answer to your questions. You may be told you are imagining things, possibly even be sent to a psychiatrist; you may be told you are just tired and need a holiday or that you have been under a lot of stress and should learn to relax. You may be given medications for some of the individual symptoms yet still find, months later, that you're feeling much the same, possibly even worse. If you've been told that it's 'all in the mind' you may even have grown to doubt your own sanity, to wonder if you really are imagining things.

This can happen when you're suffering from a symptom complex related to a cause that's not often recognized by the medical profession – if they don't ask the question 'Could it be . . . ?' they won't get an answer. There are several such causes and symptom complexes, including hypoglycaemia, allergies (particularly masked food allergies) and candidiasis. Consider the following cases.

Betty was tired, her moods were becoming erratic and, as she said, 'I've started snapping at the family and that's not like me; it's so bad that I don't blame them for being out and away from home as much as they can. I'd leave too if I could, I'm not even comfortable with myself. I'm getting fat too, I feel bloated all the time and my clothes don't fit any more, although the scales haven't changed much.' She also complained of indigestion and a bad taste in her mouth. 'I guess I do feel a bit worse round my period time, but I can't really blame it on that, for I feel out of sorts all the time, really.

June's problem had been going on for longer. Soon after she had married she had developed cystitis and she'd had several bouts since. She got indigestion in the form of flatulence and a bloated abdomen and passed so much wind she said it was embarrassing. More recently she'd started getting headaches and these had developed into migraines that occurred 'whenever the weather was warm and muggy'. Finally she said, 'TATS, I heard that used somewhere and thought, "That's me," I do feel tired all the time. Each day is an effort. I drag myself out of bed, it's a struggle to get the two boys off to school on time and my husband ready for work. Then the chores that have to be done seem endless and there's simply no time for any fun before they're all home again and I have to cook, when all I want to do is collapse in a small heap or go to bed. I eat, thinking that will give me energy, but I'm just putting on weight.'

Mark had developed bad acne as a teenager. Intermittent antibiotic treatment kept it at bay but each time he stopped the pimples returned. He found the whole business was pulling down his self-confidence. 'On top of that,' he said, 'I seem to be falling behind in class. I used to be quick and able to keep up, I was getting good grades. Now I have trouble concentrating during lessons, I can't seem to remember much of what was said and by the time I get to do my homework I feel lost. In fact I usually try and skip homework anyway, it's so difficult to concentrate, like trying to work in a fog. Trouble is, I'm now getting into trouble more, for not doing my homework and for playing up in class.'

Margaret was happily married, or, as she put it, 'We have our ups and downs like any other couple, but that's only to be expected. The trouble is, I don't seem to have any interest in sex any more, not like I used to, and I know it disappoints Tony. I suppose it's because I'm getting older. I seem to be getting PMT too, which is odd, since I haven't had it before, not in over twenty years of menstruating. On top of all that I'm not sleeping well, I get these funny pins and needles type of feelings in my legs and I feel too restless to settle down.'

James also felt that quite suddenly he was getting old. He had been a decisive quick-thinking successful businessman. Now he found he was having trouble making decisions. Whereas previously he had enjoyed the challenge of his work, he now felt overwhelmed by the responsibility. He used to work out regularly but recently he'd been getting a lot of vague aches and pains in his muscles. The thought that this was middle age creeping up depressed him, and to cap it all he was getting 'old man's syndrome' as he called it, the symptoms of prostatitis. He was drinking more too, finding that whereas he had been a purely social drinker he now longed for lunch when he could go to the pub and have a few beers and a sandwich, even if it did cause indigestion and bloating afterwards. He was also getting more hangovers. 'I know I'm drinking a bit more, but not that much, I used to have a good "head", I used not to get a hangover unless I really drank a lot, now I wake up with one most mornings.'

Imagine what would happen if any of these individuals went to a doctor who was not thinking of candidiasis. Betty would be told, 'It's just normal, you're doing too much, learn to relax, have a holiday and you'll feel fine.' June would be given an antibiotic for the cystitis, thus worsening her symptoms, and another drug for her migraines. Mark might be sent for counselling. Margaret would be given a sleeping pill and James treated for incipient alcoholism.

In fact they are *all* examples of candidiasis, the complex of symptoms that can develop when *Candida albicans*, a type of mould or yeast, becomes dominant in different cavities within the body, especially the digestive tract and the genito-urinary system. The problem, and particularly its consequences, can then spread from there and affect almost every aspect of the body and of the emotions.

CHAPTER 2

Self-diagnosis

So you think you, or someone you know, has candidiasis. Listed below are some of the many possible symptoms. By checking your symptoms against this list, you will be able to make a probable diagnosis for yourself. If you follow the diet and take the supplements explained in this book, you can probably solve the problem on your own. Many people have done so and many will continue to do so.

Symptom list

The following is a list of symptoms that can occur in candidiasis. They do not all necessarily indicate candidiasis; there could be other reasons for some or all of them. However, the more of them you have, the more likely it is that candidiasis is your problem.

General symptoms
Fatigue and lethargy
Insomnia
Drowsiness
Poor coordination
History of ringworm or other fungal infection of the skin
Body odour, even after washing
Ear infections

Mental symptoms
Confusion
Poor memory

Poor concentration
Irritability
Anxiety
Mood swings
Crying without apparent cause
Feeling spacy or as if in a fog
Poor decision making
Headaches

Digestive symptoms
White-coated tongue
Bad breath
Sore mouth
Frequent sore throats
Gas and burping
Bloating and flatulence
Diarrhoea
Constipation
Alternating diarrhoea and constipation
White discharge from the bowels
Rectal itch

Diet symptoms
Cravings for bread, cheese or sugar
A preferred diet containing many of the forbidden foods (see list)
Increasing consumption of and craving for alcoholic drinks
Sensitivity to certain foods

Genito-urinary symptoms
Vaginal itch or burning
Vaginal discharge (white or creamy)
Repeating 'cystitis', unresponsive to antibiotics (long term)
Premenstrual tension
Painful periods
Menstrual cramps
Decreased interest in sexual activity

Infertility
Prostatitis
Impotence

Respiratory system symptoms
Sinus congestion and catarrh
Post-nasal drip
Mucus in throat

Symptoms in the limbs
Fungal infection under the fingernails
Fungal infection between the toes ('athlete's foot')
Muscle weakness
Muscle pains
Joint swelling
Joint pains

Symptoms in your medical history
Frequent use of antibiotics
Taking the contraceptive pill
Use of steroid drugs such as cortisone or prednisone
Symptoms made worse by damp, humid weather
Feel worse in dank or mouldy environments
Increased sensitivity to chemicals and pollutants

Based on the above list of symptoms you may think that you have candidiasis. If you have made the right diagnosis, and if your condition responds to the treatment suggested in this book, you will have saved yourself a lot of problems (a) by eliminating the problem itself and (b) by avoiding the various side-tracks that you can be taken down by practitioners unfamiliar with the problem, its diagnosis and its treatment.

If your self-diagnosis is wrong, and candidiasis is not your problem, you won't have done yourself any harm. The treatment is not only safe, it's actually beneficial for everybody because it encourages you to avoid sugar, sweet foods, white flour, and other refined carbohydrates, and to reduce alcohol intake. However, if your symptoms do not respond to treatment then it's wise to see a practitioner. You may have some other problem, or your candidiasis treatment may need some guidance.

In these cases, generally the best person to visit is a naturopath (natural therapist). Naturopaths are usually well trained in the recognition, detection and treatment of systemic candidiasis. They will almost certainly take an extensive history, they will probably ask you unexpected questions, ones you may not have been asked before when visiting a doctor with the current problem. Few people, for instance, when complaining of mood swings, irritability, bloating and indigestion, are asked if they are on the contraceptive pill or if bread and cheese are favourite foods. It is essential that you tell the practitioner *everything*. Candidiasis is treatable, but it is not necessarily a simple problem, nor is it always amenable to a simple or single solution.

FAILURE TO DIAGNOSE

It is all too easy to fail to diagnose candidiasis correctly. You may even unwittingly contribute to this failure yourself by trying to avoid the diagnosis because you have heard of some of the dietary restrictions that will be necessary if candidiasis is confirmed. I've often heard a patient say, 'Oh, please don't tell me I have candida; I hate the thought of the diet I'll have to go on. Can't we look for something else first?' In one extreme case my receptionist told me that a patient had left, saying, 'I'm going to find another practitioner – one who won't tell me that I have candida and have to give up all those foods.' Sadly, by the time I saw that patient again, many months later, her condition was much worse. However, by then she was willing to embark on the correct treatment and soon had the problem solved.

It is particularly uncommon for doctors to diagnose candidiasis. Following the appropriate testing and swabs they may diagnose vaginal thrush or oral thrush. However, they rarely consider the possibility that candida can be a systemic problem or recognize that candida overgrowth in the digestive tract can lead to a wide range of physical symptoms throughout the body, as well as behavioural and mood changes.

In cases of suspected candidiasis the best person to visit is a naturopath or natural therapist. Naturopaths are usually well-trained in the recognition, detection and treatment of systemic candidiasis. They will almost certainly take an extensive history, ask you unexpected questions and come up with an explanation that covers many of your problems.

If you do think that you may have candidiasis, face up to the treatment described in this book and give it a go. If this fails to resolve the problem you absolutely must seek further professional guidance. If you do not, the symptoms will worsen and could wreck havoc with your life. When I started in practice, twenty or more years ago, public awareness was rare: few people had heard of candidiasis and fewer still knew what to do about it. Now the story is different and help should be easy to find; so face up to your problem and get rid of it. It's well worth every effort.

> Margaret came to see me with a variety of problems. 'Emotionally I'm a mess,' she said. 'I used to be alert and self-confident. I had a local part-time job, looked after the house and children, and entertained with my husband as part of his work. It was hectic but I coped and enjoyed it. I was also looking forward to going back to my old job full time. I was slim, I looked good and we were a happy family.'
>
> 'So what happened?' I asked.
>
> 'I don't know. I did go back to work but I found I couldn't do the things I used to do. It was as if my brain had been turned off, gone fuzzy. I started to forget things, got confused, couldn't concentrate – and my work was very demanding. I put it down to years away from my profession, but I don't know . . . It's been four years now and things are getting worse, not better. One minute I'm happy, the next I'm in tears for no reason. I snap at the kids. I don't enjoy entertaining any more: wine gives me a headache and no matter what I eat I get dreadful indigestion. Somehow everything seems to have gone wrong.'
>
> A few more questions from me, a couple of tests and I was sure that her problem was systemic candidiasis. A change of diet, a few supplements (as discussed further on) and in no time at all Margaret

was saying: 'It's as if a fog had been lifted from my brain and stabilizers added to my emotions. No more headaches or indigestion – it's wonderful! I can entertain, enjoy the company of my friends and family, and feel in control of my job – and enjoy that too!'

Poor Margaret had suffered needlessly for years. As she admitted, the changes in her diet were a nuisance but the benefits were more than worth it.

Since the diagnosis of candidiasis is often difficult, ultimately the correct diagnosis may lie with the cure. If the cure for a particular illness makes you feel better, then that's the illness you've had. This means that if you have tried more or less 'everything' but are still suffering, if you cannot get a definitive diagnosis but suspect that candidiasis could be your problem, you should try the treatment described in these pages. If nothing else, as has been seen time and again, this treatment will improve your general health and well-being. If you are suffering from candidiasis, it will, when properly managed, relieve that problem too.

CHAPTER 3

A Definition of Candida

Let's find out how candida fits into the natural world. There is a major group of species grouped together under the name of fungi. For a long time they were considered to belong to the botanical kingdom Plantae, or plants. However, they do not have chlorophyl, the green pigment in leaves by which plants can turn air and water into carbohydrates which provide both energy and the raw materials for the plant's structure; many don't have roots to anchor them in place and provide pathways up which nutrients, including water, can be drawn. For these and related reasons they are now generally considered as a botanical kingdom of their own.

There are many different types of fungi, possibly a hundred thousand or more, including yeasts, moulds, mushrooms, truffles, rusts and smuts. Within the yeast group there are several hundred types, one of which is the group of candida organisms. The major one with which we are dealing here is *Candida albicans*. Other types of yeast include those used in brewing, bread baking and in fermenting dairy products.

Our world is inhabited by a wide range of yeasts, bacteria and protozoa. Millions of them live in and on the human body, millions more live in homes, gardens and the rest of your environment. Provided a correct and healthy balance is maintained, many of them do you no harm, and many, like the yeasts used to make wine and beer and the bacteria and other organisms that are a constructive part of your digestive system, are highly beneficial. However, there are yeasts that do cause problems. They include *Aspergillus*, which commonly infects the tonsils and much of the respiratory tract, and *Trichophyton*, which, when active between the toes, causes the condition commonly referred to as 'athlete's foot' as it breeds particularly well in warm, dark and moist crevices. *Candida albicans* normally inhabits the skin, and the mucous membranes of the digestive tract, respiratory tract and vagina, but only in relatively small numbers.

This is not the place for a detailed discussion of the biochemistry and physiology of candidiasis. However it has been my experience, in practice, that patients stick to their treatment programme better if they have some knowledge of what is happening. So here is a simple outline.

Candida albicans colonizes the human digestive tract, usually within a few months of birth. When it is present in small numbers, and in balance with all the other organisms within the digestive tract, it does little or no harm. The problem comes when its numbers grow and it becomes dominant. In addition, if it is not well fed it can change into a mould form and become more aggressive in the way it gets its nourishment. This involves attaching itself to surfaces and then secreting enzymes which damage them and dissolve them until individual molecules can be absorbed. You can think of this as a type of external digestive process. If this is small-scale little harm is done, even if it is the lining of your digestive tract that's being damaged, since the surface cells are naturally dying, falling off and being replaced from below at an extremely rapid rate. The problems come when the yeast's numbers grow and the damage increases and becomes invasive: the main ones are the physical damage to the gut wall and its consequences, commonly referred to as 'leaky gut syndrome'; the consequences of the toxic chemicals the yeasts produce; and their excessive numbers disadvantaging other types of organisms, many of which are beneficial to you, the host.

Let's consider the leaky gut syndrome first. As a result of the damage to the mucosal membranes, partially digested food can leak through the damaged portions and enter the bloodstream as large molecules. Your ever-vigilant immune system recognizes these proteins as foreign substances and sets up a reaction to them. In this way food intolerances are created, sometimes called food allergies although this latter term is not strictly correct. Whenever you eat these foods you will get a reaction; unfortunately it is a masked reaction, not obvious in the way that a true allergic reaction is, and so much more difficult to detect. Yet they may be making a major contribution to your symptoms: general lethargy, mood changes, frequent headaches, dermatitis, asthma, arthritis and others. The reactions are prolonged and are with you most of the time, and as the damage caused by the candida continues and increases the number of the offending foods may well be growing. The leaky gut problem can also contribute to your malnutrition. Many essential nutrients will not be absorbed since they require transport molecules to act, and these are normally part of the healthy cells lining the mucosal membranes of your digestive tract. When candida damages these proper routes of absorption, essential nutrients continue along the digestive system and are excreted.

The cells lining your digestive tract produce digestive enzymes. If these cells are damaged the enzymes are not produced, and so carbohydrates, particularly the disaccharides such as maltose (from grains), lactose (from milk) and sucrose (table sugar), are not broken down and digested but build up in the small intestine, and this can lead to diarrhoea. They can also act as food for the candida and encourage its growth.

Many of the chemicals released by the candida are toxic to you, the host – they're meant to be, since this is how the candida gets its nourishment, as we have seen. As well as damaging you locally, they can enter your bloodstream, travel throughout your body and cause a variety of unpleasant physical symptoms. Some of these chemicals are alcohols, often produced in considerable quantities. When they reach your liver they are transformed by oxidation into aldehydes, which in turn produce hangover-type symptoms. In fact many people suffering from candidiasis report feeling drunk even if they have not been drinking alcohol, and one patient was even reported on a drink-driving charge – though he was a teetotaller. Candida can also cause emotional symptoms including mood swings, anxiety, irritability and depression.

When candida becomes dominant it can crowd out beneficial organisms, including the bacteria that produce nutrients you need. These nutrients include several of the B-group vitamins, biotin and vitamin K, and this contributes to your malnutrition. Also, the altered chemistry it produces can result in the environment within your intestines changing, and in a way that allows a variety of other unwanted pathogens to become dominant species, creating further health problems.

If the damage occurs in the duodenum and small intestine the full range of consequences can develop. If it occurs in the respiratory system, in the digestive tract above the stomach (namely, the mouth, throat and oesophagus), or in the genito-urinary tract the consequences will be similar but localized; you will be more likely to see and be aware of the dead cells coming away, accompanied by the secreted mucus, the creamy discharge your cells have produced in an effort to wash away the organisms. This mucus is an obvious symptom of thrush.

For a few sufferers, in whom the problem is not treated or develops further, the symptoms may become even more severe, and the candida organisms in the digestive tract themselves enter the bloodstream through the leaky gut and travel throughout the body where they can continue to do damage. The digestive tract, the respiratory system and the genito-urinary tract are cavities within the total space occupied by your body. A solid object placed inside your mouth is not actually 'inside' your body, although it is 'within its space': no barrier has been passed; no skin or mucosal membrane has been crossed. When candida damages one of these cavities the problem is serious; but once it has passed through the skin or across the mucosal membranes lining your digestive tract and entered the bloodstream, it is truly *inside* your body, and the harm it can do is a lot greater and its expulsion is a great deal more difficult. This is a serious situation and strenuous efforts should be made to avoid it. If it has already occurred it is essential that professional help is obtained. If in addition to absorbing the candida organisms you become allergic to them, the range of possible symptoms and consequences is unlimited.

From this discussion I hope you will understand how important it is to treat the problem the moment it is recognized. I have heard patients say, 'It's all too much effort, I really can't be bothered, it's not so bad that I can't live with it.' It may not be that bad now, but if you do nothing it will almost certainly get worse – and the worse it gets the harder it is to treat and the more serious the consequences.

CHAPTER 4

Secondary Problems

There are many secondary problems that result from the presence of *Candida albicans*, all of them typical, all of them commonly misdiagnosed and all of them causing, or having the power to cause, havoc in the lives not only of the individuals concerned but in those around them. Let's look at a few examples.

CYSTITIS

Many women suffer from this annoying, painful and often recurrent problem. They experience pain and burning on urinating coupled with an increased urgency and need to 'go', and yet when they do go there may be very little urine to pass. The apparent cause of the problem is a bacterial infection that has invaded the bladder. The usual treatment is antibiotics. However, the condition can be a lot more complicated than that.

After the first infection and treatment with an antibiotic the bacteria may have been killed, but not the moulds or yeasts that are also present. In addition the local tissues have not been healed. This is all the chance that *Candida albicans* needs. It has survived, the competing bacteria have been killed, there is empty space and it can take over, multiply and become a dominant organism. Thrush then develops with its typical itch and white cheesy discharge. This further damages the tissues of the bladder and vagina leaving the ideal environment for new bacteria to colonize, and so cystitis develops yet again. When further antibiotic treatment is given the cycle is repeated. If no one recognizes that the real problem is the candidiasis then this cycle will be repeated, not once but many times. There is also the danger that the increasing number of candida cells can spread and invade the digestive tract and other body cavities. The solution is not more antibiotics, it is fighting the candida and repairing the damage.

DIGESTIVE PROBLEMS

Candida can affect the entire length of the digestive tract. If you have taken antibiotics the scenario can be much like that in the genito-urinary tract in the case of cystitis.

Susan had taken several courses of antibiotics prescribed when she had flu. These had done little to help her fight the flu, as it's caused by a virus, not bacteria. A virus, not being a living organism, cannot be killed and is therefore not harmed by an antibiotic. The antibiotics *had* killed off a large proportion of the beneficial bacteria in the digestive tract, as well as any unwanted or toxic bacteria that might have been lurking there, but they did no harm to the small amounts of moulds that are always there. The space left as a result gave the candida the chance to multiply and spread. (Note, within a few months of birth some candida organisms are present in everyone but they are too few to cause problems.)

She then experienced a variety of mild digestive problems. She started to feel bloated, especially after snacking on sweets or dried fruit, eating sandwiches or drinking wine, all foods that encourage the growth of moulds. She passed wind, started to burp and experienced a feeling of fullness after meals. Her tongue had a white coating and she said she was beginning to get bad breath and had had frequent sore throats recently, in fact she was thinking of going to the doctor to get yet another antibiotic.

Had she done this she would have only have encouraged the candida further. In her case it had started in the small intestine, then spread throughout the lower digestive tract, into the stomach, up the oesophagus and on to the throat and tongue. The solution was not more antibiotics, it was to fight the candida and restore both normal gut flora and the normal activity of the digestive tract.

Rosemary had similar symptoms but in her case they came on after she had cystitis which was treated with antibiotics and developed into thrush. Because of the shape of the female anatomy it is very easy for the moulds to migrate from the vagina back to the anus and up into the digestive system. From then on the scenario was much the same as in Susan's case. Again the solution was not to treat the cystitis with antibiotics or treat the digestive upsets with antacids as she had been doing, it was to fight the candida and restore the normal environment.

'FEMALE' PROBLEMS

Yvette started using the contraceptive pill. Soon after that she began to experience PMT in the form of bloating and swollen breasts each month plus emotional problems. Initially it was an overall sense of irritability, of being easily irritated, snapping at friends and family and generally being on a short fuse. In time this developed into a pattern of wild mood swings, occurring all the time, not just in the few days leading up to her period. One minute she was wildly happy, bubbling and sparkling; then she would slump into deep depression and find herself crying for no particular reason; in between she said she would often burst into tears at the slightest thing, a mild criticism, small frustration or even for no reason at all. Her doctor had suggested an antidepressant but that was not the answer. The answer was to stop taking the contraceptive pill, and treat the candida, which can develop in many women when they take the pill.

Once the underlying problem has been diagnosed as candidiasis, that's what should be treated, not the consequences. Too often I hear patients saying, even after I have explained the full treatment, 'Yes, but in the meantime, could you give me something specifically for the bloating and wind, something for the mood swings, for the headaches or for the cystitis?' There is little point in doing so as the cause, the overgrowth of candida, will still be there. Many of the food sensitivities exist because of the damage to the gut wall and the depression of the immune system. The hypoglycaemia is there because of the effect of candida on the adrenal glands and the body's incapacity to maintain normal blood-sugar levels; the headaches result from the erratic blood-sugar levels, the induced sensitivities or from the effect of toxic compounds released both by the candida and as a result of the body's attempts to deal with these compounds, and the cystitis is a consequence of the damage done by the candida to the bladder lining.

Solve the initial and primary causative problem, the presence of *Candida albicans*, even though it may take a little while, and the gut will heal, the immune system will have a chance to recover, the blood-sugar level will normalize, brain chemistry will improve and cystitis will stop as the bladder recovers.

PART TWO

Treatment

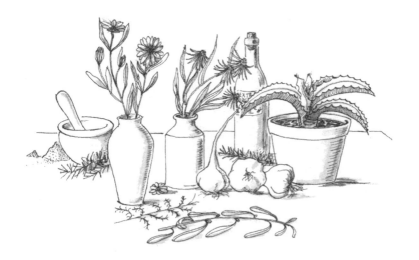

CHAPTER 5

Diet

Before we start it is important to mention that there is no single treatment for candidiasis. You, as an individual, will have your own specific needs. You may need to follow a very strict diet indeed, eating only protein-rich foods, nuts and vegetables, and keeping the total carbohydrate content down. Alternatively some extra carbohydrate may not cause problems and this may mean you can include grains as well. If the problem is even less severe you may be able to include fresh fruit. It's the same with the supplements mentioned below. You may need all of them or, more commonly, you may need just some. If you are working on your own you will have to experiment. A good starting point is to change your diet to eliminate only the foods listed below. If you are working with a practitioner then they will be able to advise you on any finer points applicable to you.

CANDIDIASIS, FOOD, AND FOOD INTOLERANCE

For anyone with candidiasis there are certain foods you should definitely avoid. These are ones that contain yeasts, are made by a fermentation process or, like dried fruits, are likely to carry yeasts on their surfaces. You should also avoid all sugars and all sugar-rich foods. In addition, if you have developed food intolerances you will also have to avoid those foods. In general you will need someone else to help you identify these but, to eliminate the possibility of addiction, you might be wise to begin by avoiding the foods you love or choose to eat every day. Unfortunately, though not coincidentally, these yeast-based and sugar-rich foods will often have come to occupy a major position in your diet. When you've read the list you may find yourself thinking, 'But that's nearly everything I eat,' and, 'I couldn't give up *those* foods, they're my favourites,' or, 'They're the ones I crave.' If so it is particularly important that you *do* go without them. People with candidiasis commonly do eat a lot of these foods. It's a bit of a chicken-and-egg situation: you may never find out if you have developed candidiasis so readily because of your high intake of yeast-based foods or if it was the development of candidiasis that gave you the urge to change your eating pattern and eat an increasing amount of these yeast-based foods.

Fortunately the problem is now well recognized, and there are many specialized yeast-free products. Health-food shops are an excellent source. It's also becoming easier to find out the ingredients within a particular package or tin. Many people manage to control their diet while eating at home where they either prepare the food for themselves or have it prepared for them by someone who fully understands the rules. Fewer people are successful in negotiating the pitfalls when eating out, either in restaurants or with friends and family. Through fear of causing or experiencing embarrassment you may decide to forgo your diet on social occasions and suffer the consequences. Learning what to say and how to cope in these situations is an invaluable part of dealing with the problem successfully and not taking one step backwards for every two you take forwards. It is also simple to do, once you get the hang of it, as you are about to find out in Part 3.

Many foods that cause you problems, either because of candidiasis or because of allergies and food intolerances you have developed, have also become addictive. You actually become addicted to the foods that are doing you harm. This is a crucial point when considering food intolerances and so is worth explaining.

Throughout a healthy body there are cells that have 'receptor sites', specialized areas of the cell membrane that respond to specific chemicals as they circulate through your bloodstream. The brain has receptors that respond to opiates, morphine and morphine-related compounds, and these are concentrated in the areas that control pain awareness. When these opiates are taken up by your brain pain is controlled and the feeling of well-being increases. Food addiction can replicate this natural process.

Proteins occur in the body and in food. They are long chains made up of hundreds of individual amino acid molecules. During protein digestion these very large molecules are broken down into much smaller ones, chains of amino acids from as short as two or three amino acids to twenty or more, and these shorter chains are called peptides. During *normal* digestion, the peptides are broken down further, into individual amino acids, which are then absorbed. However, in candidiasis, when a leaky gut occurs it is these peptides that are absorbed, and some of them will be the specific sequence of amino acids that act on the brain's opiate receptors. They produce a high, made up of reduced pain and increased well-being, an effect like morphine. It is this to which you can become addicted.

Put simply, once you become intolerant of a certain food, every time you eat that food it gives you a chemical high. But soon afterwards the effect wears off and you feel let down. At this point you start to want that food (and its effect) all over again; you crave it and feel you simply *have* to eat it. So the cycle repeats itself. Furthermore, because the foods are often ones that you consider good for you, such as bread or milk, you feel that it's simply your body telling you that you need them and that it is right that you should eat them. This can make it all the harder for you to understand that you should *not*. I have seen grown men cry when given the list of foods they must avoid, simply because the craving is so strong.

Foods to Avoid at All Costs

- Bread, buns, pizzas, yeasted cakes, doughnuts and any other food made with yeast as the raising agent
- Fermented grain products such as soda bread (it contains soured milk) and pumpernickel bread

- 'Yeast-free' breads commonly do contain yeasts and related organisms as the dough is allowed to 'sit' for a while, commonly in a bakery in vats open to the yeast-laden air, and 'ferment'. A variety of compounds and gases form in the dough and these provide much of the texture and flavour
- Cheese, yogurt, soured and fermented dairy products
- Alcohol (with the possible exception of neat spirits)
- Vinegar; mayonnaise, salad dressings and any other food containing vinegar
- Pickles and olives
- Tinned tomatoes
- Tomato products such as juice, sauce, purée and paste
- Soya sauce, and most other similar sauces if any of the ingredients have been fermented or include vinegar
- Marmite and similar yeast-based spreads
- Mushrooms
- Smoked foods such as kippers, bacon, ham and smoked cheeses
- Malt
- Dried fruit
- Melons, fresh or dried
- Fruit juices, cordials and soft drinks
- Tinned fruits or commercially preserved fruits
- Desiccated coconut and other coconut products
- Peanuts, peanut butter and any other peanut products
- Dried herbs
- Pasteurized milk should be avoided both because of the sugar it contains (lactose) and because it encourages the growth of candida. Cream is less of a problem, but it is high in fat
- Sugar in any form including table sugar, honey, syrup, rice sugar

If your problem is severe you may have to avoid all fruit. Initially it would be wise to limit your intake of fruit and, where possible, select vegetables instead.

Some Basic Alternatives

- Alcohol: neat spirits are a possible exception
- Vinegar: fresh lemon juice
- Tomato products: fresh tomatoes
- Dried herbs: fresh herbs. Spices are generally safe
- Milk: see pages 51–2

If your problem is severe and if it doesn't respond to the initial treatment program, you may even have to reduce your intake of grains, and rely on protein foods and vegetables for a while. You can experiment with this for yourself.

SUPPLEMENTS, HERBS AND OTHER REMEDIES

Many substances can help to control both the extensive growth of the organism and the form in which it occurs. These include supplements (vitamins, minerals, amino acids and other nutritional substances), herbs (including foods such as garlic) and homoeopathic and flower remedies. Since candidiasis takes such varied forms you will need to determine which ones will be of particular benefit to you, and also to determine how much you should take. Any quantities given below are at best a guideline; your own specific requirements may be different.

1 To improve the intestinal environment in such a way that candida growth is limited
- Hydrochloric acid, in tablet form. Most people with candidiasis have a reduced ability to produce hydrochloric acid, naturally present in the stomach. A supplement should be taken but only at the end of meals. This allows the food and saliva to stimulate the maximum production of acid of which your stomach is capable, and which will digest the first part of the meal, and the supplement will help with the rest.

- Digestive enzymes for the stomach and the intestines. These are required to ensure a minimal amount of undigested food is left available for the candida to live on.
- Fibre supplements and a high-fibre diet. Strictly speaking, 'fibre' is 'non-digestible carbohydrate'. This non-digestible carbohydrate *may* be fibrous, as in the case of the fibres in celery and many other vegetables, or it may not be, such as the 'fibre' (non-digestible carbohydrates) found in food such as linseeds, slippery elm powder, psyllium hulls and grain brans (oat bran; corn bran; wheat bran, rice bran etc). The aim is to ensure the normal, rapid transit of waste matter through the digestive tract. They do this by adding bulk to the stool. This is further increased by the water they take up and absorb. They also take up, or absorb, a number of the toxins produced by the candida, as well as the organisms themselves, both alive and dead.

2   *To kill the candida and other unwanted organisms*

- Propolis tincture. This is the substance made by bees that inhibits mould growth in their hives.
- Caprylic acid, a fatty acid that inhibits fungal growth.
- Garlic. Garlic is anti-fungal and can be taken in capsule form. However, the important compounds it contains are easily damaged and the best results are usually obtained with fresh garlic, which should be eaten as often as possible. Don't use the odourless forms of garlic as many of the active ingredients are also removed during the process of removing the odour. Garlic can also be obtained in freeze-dried form.
- Anti-fungal herbs include echinacea, eucalyptus, golden seal, marigold and myrrh.
- Useful homoeopathic remedies include silicea and thuja.
- Grapefruit seed extract is anti-bacterial and anti-fungal; it is also active against parasites in general. It can be taken in liquid or capsule form.
- Biotin inhibits the conversion of *Candida albicans* to its more harmful fungal form.

- Olive oil should be used in all cooking and salads. It is rich in a fatty acid called oleic acid that also inhibits the conversion of *Candida albicans* to the fungal form.

3 To increase the strength and integrity of the intestinal walls, to limit the damage being done and to reduce the effect of existing allergies and intolerances, and to prevent the formation of new ones

- Slippery elm powder. This coats and protects the mucosal membranes. It should be taken regularly until any damaged area is healed. 1 teaspoonful twice a day is normally sufficient. It can be mashed into banana (in which form it seems to be readily acceptable) unless you are avoiding all fruits, or mixed with any other food. In liquids it may go lumpy. Do not use 'slippery elm food', which is only 2 per cent slippery elm powder; you must get the 100 per cent pure form.
- Aloe vera juice. 50 ml of the fresh juice (less if concentrated) taken three times a day improves the healing of any damaged area of intestinal walls. It is also thought to have some anti-fungal action.
- Vitamins A and E; coenzyme Q10; zinc; the amino acid derivative glutamine and gama-oryzanol, obtained from rice bran. These all improve the healing of the digestive tract and help to reduce the risk of further damage.

4 To provide organisms that compete with candida albicans and thus help to contain it and repopulate the intestines
These can be started about a week after the anti-fungals, when the toxins from the die-off effect are diminishing.

- *Lactobacillus acidophilus*, *Bifidus* and related organisms. These are available as tablets or in powdered form, some of which are not stable unless kept under refrigeration.
- FOS, fructo-oligosaccharides. Two of these, inulin and oligo-fructose, are particularly important. They are sugars (saccharides), found in vegetables, but unlike table sugar (sucrose) and honey (fructose and glucose) they do not stimulate the production of

yeasts. They act as nutrient sources for the beneficial organisms, particularly the bifidobacteria *Bifidus* and *Lactobacillus acidophilus*, and have been shown to increase their numbers tenfold. Inulin is also converted in the colon into the short-chain fatty acids that are used for energy and repair by the walls of the small intestine and colon. In addition they have an antibiotic-like effect.

- NAG (N-Acetyl-D-Glucosamine). This protects the intestinal walls. It improves the ability of the beneficial organisms, such as bifidobacteria, to attach, while at the same time inhibiting the attachment of *Candida albicans*.

5 To treat the genito-urinary tract
Women should douche and men wash with a combination of the following once or twice a day, or when the symptoms create discomfort: fresh aloe vera juice, 100ml (if using a concentrate, dilute as indicated); propolis tincture, 5–10 drops; grapefruit seed extract, 5–10 drops. Women should also apply aloe vera gel as far internally as possible in between times or insert one or two capsules of *Lactobacillus acidophilus*.

6 To improve and strengthen the normal functioning of the immune system
- A general multi-vitamin and multi-mineral supplement containing all the essential trace nutrients, taken as directed.
- Additional amounts of anti-oxidants including vitamin A and beta-carotene, vitamin C, the bioflavonoids and OPCs, zinc, manganese, selenium.

7 To handle specific symptoms, physical and emotional, related to your individual situation
Emotional problems will respond as the candidiasis is brought under control. However, in the meantime, flower remedies can help and there are many excellent books to help you choose the appropriate ones. Other treatments can be recommended by your practitioner. However, keep in mind that candida can cause a wide range of symptoms, and simply solving this root problem can

resolve other problems you currently have. If you feel that you're doing everything that has been recommended and the candidiasis is still resisting treatment it is possible that parasites are compounding the problem. You will need the help of a practitioner to establish this.

CHAPTER 6

Lifestyle

Treating candidiasis successfully involves your total lifestyle.

You have already seen the list of foods that you must avoid. Part 3 will not only provide you with specific recipes; it will also give you a number of suggestions for dealing with food and eating in a variety of situations, such as socially with friends, in restaurants and on the run.

The treatment also involves what you wear. Moulds love warm, damp, dark spaces with limited airflow. If you are a woman you should stop wearing pantyhose or tights and swap them for old-fashioned stockings. Do not wear pants made of nylon or other artificial materials, choose cotton underwear instead. Wear skirts rather than trousers or slacks; if you must wear trousers, choose ones that are very loose. Men should wear cotton underwear and loose trousers rather than tight jeans.

Your sexual activities also deserve some thought. If you have a regular partner it is likely that they too will have the problem. Just as you douched or washed with a combination of aloe vera juice, propolis tincture and grapefruit seed extract, so should they. It is important that you both become clear or the opportunity for re-infection exists. If you do not have a regular sexual partner you should be aware that you can infect any casual partner you have and that they can reinfect you. If you have recently had thrush and feel you are just getting your health back, the chances are high that you are particularly vulnerable to picking it up again.

Your environment is also important. You should avoid damp environments where airborne moulds are ever-present. Your bedclothes should be cotton or linen sheets rather than synthetic.

Avoid electric blankets and keep the windows open at night to ensure circulating fresh air. Air-conditioning is also inadvisable.

Your emotional state is fundamental. Candidiasis can bring rapid emotional swings, alternating highs and lows, sudden irritability and equally sudden tears and depression. All these moods and changes can occur without apparent reason. Since they are largely caused by the chemical effects of the candida, the solution is to resolve the candida.

However, if you do already have emotional problems in relation to specific issues, then by working on them and resolving them you can create a more stable emotional balance and be less likely to be affected by the chemical disturbances. In addition, you may benefit from help in dealing with these mood swings and the problems they can create in your relationships with the people around you. For these reasons, some outside help, in the form of counselling, psychotherapy or other emotional treatment therapies may be beneficial.

CHAPTER 7

Coping with the Treatment

The treatment involves radical changes in diet and lifestyle, and can pose its own problems. In this section we are going to look at ways to minimize these disruptions. There are many different ways of coping with the dietary restrictions, the supplements and the lifestyle changes. The ones you choose will depend not only on your own personal choice but on your lifestyle and whether you live on your own or with other people. Some people choose to make a clean sweep of the kitchen, others partition it so that the foods they can't eat are in a separate section. Some people like to find alternatives to forbidden foods, others like to discover what entirely new eating styles they can develop out of their permitted foods.

Some people like to start making the dietary changes gradually, but in general this is a poor idea. By cutting out 90 per cent of the offending foods you may only make a small difference to the organisms present and to your symptoms. By making that extra effort, by avoiding the other 10 per cent, you may find you are making a dramatic difference and suddenly feel that the effort is worthwhile.

Some people start the treatment full of enthusiasm and stick to it for a few weeks, then get disheartened and give up; or else they are faced with a social situation and decide to forget it all and have a good time, promising themselves they will start the treatment again later. The danger with this stop–start approach is that when you start you probably kill off the weaker organisms, then when you stop the stronger ones are left and can proliferate. When you start again you're left with a population based on the tougher and more resistant organisms and these are obviously more difficult to deal with than the original mixed population. All this means that you may find it is more difficult to get positive results from the treatment the second time around. It's much better to start the treatment and see it through to the end. Ultimately this takes less time and is usually easier than the stop–start approach.

No one will pretend that the treatment is easy. It's not simply a case of avoiding one or two foods: many people find that a large part of their diet is made up of or contains foods or components that are no longer permitted. If you live alone then eating at home is relatively simple since you are in charge of the kitchen and can control what is available (as temptations) as well as what is used. It's much easier to stay on the diet if you have eliminated the forbidden foods from your kitchen than if you have to face them daily and resist the temptation to eat them.

If you live with other people, try to enlist their support – after all, anyone can fall prey to candidiasis, and a spell without the yeast-encouraging foods could be good for everyone. Even if they don't stick to the eating plan as rigorously as you must, the less food you have in the house to tempt you the better, and so each limitation on their part is a help.

If the people at home insist on eating cheese sandwiches and bringing home a pizza, about the worst meals you could face if you have candidiasis, then do try to get their agreement that the meals you eat together can be shared, or at least the main dishes. If, for instance, they want mushrooms in the casserole, perhaps you can persuade them instead to do a mushroom-free casserole that you and they can share, and have a mushroom dish on the side for themselves.

Eating meals away from home, unless you have prepared them and taken them with you, is even more difficult. Here the problem is threefold. You have the frustration of struggling to find things you can eat, the sense of deprivation at having to forgo many tempting dishes that you would love to eat, and the possible discomfort or embarrassment you may feel if other people are present and either become aware of or get involved in the problem.

Even drinking can become a problem and this has many social implications with which you have to deal.

In general, the solution is up to you. Look at it this way. You do have candidiasis, and that's no fun. The symptoms are unpleasant, and if you do not deal with the situation then it will get worse. At best they will linger on, adversely affecting your life in a variety of ways, both overt and covert, major and minor. Since there is a solution, now is the time to embrace it. Be thankful that something can be done. Take the positive view that you are on the road back to recovery and full health.

Look on this as a time to explore new culinary delights and new taste sensations, and to do some interesting experiments in and around the kitchen. Talk positively, not negatively. If you moan, others will moan with you; they will probably also try to tempt you off the diet, saying that a small amount of this and that can't hurt whereas you know, of course, that it can. If on the other hand you indicate that there is no problem, that you don't mind going without this and that food or drink for a while, then they will soon forget about it and assume you are having as good a time as they are. There is no need to be embarrassed. If you were diabetic it would be simple to say 'Sorry, I don't eat sugar or sweet things', and no one would comment. You can do the same with this diet.

So summon up your inner resources, focus on the benefits you will be getting and look for additional benefits like improvement in your skin and hair and overall health, plus increased energy.

Weight Loss

If you would like to lose weight this is an excellent time. There are so many foods you must avoid that are fattening, such as sugar, bread and cheese, to say nothing of the calories you will avoid by not drinking beer or wine, that you could find yourself simply eating less and losing weight as a result of the dietary restrictions imposed here. This is particularly true if you are slow to find alternative foods and drinks that you can eat.

If on the other hand you don't want to lose weight, you'll find a wide variety of alternative foods and recipe suggestions in the next section and you should make a particular effort to stock up on permitted foods, including raw nuts and seeds.

THE DIE-OFF EFFECT

There is, when you first experience it, little so frustrating and disheartening as making the effort to follow the treatment, down to the finest detail, and then finding that you're not only getting worse but that some new symptoms are developing – increased bloating, an upset stomach, diarrhoea or constipation, headaches, a coated tongue or a sore throat, an increase of mucus or phlegm or a worsening of many of your other symptoms and, in fact, almost any of the symptoms already listed. This does not always happen, but when it does it's the 'die-off effect'.

Do not despair. It may not be much fun, but it is proof that the treatment is working. It also tells you that the treatment is necessary and that it is important that you continue. Let me explain what is happening.

It is important that you understand that there is nothing in the treatment that would cause these symptoms to occur if you were totally healthy to start with. They occur as a result of the effect of the treatment on the *Candida albicans* present in your digestive tract. Some of them come about due to the changes you are making in your digestive tract, such as increased acidity and more enzymes. There is also the effect of the organisms you are sending down. You could liken it to microbial warfare. The good ones fight the bad ones and produce a range of gases and chemicals. On top of that, when the cells of *Candida albicans* die chemicals are released, not slowly, as they were when you had the problem, but suddenly, as the death rate of the candida cells rises.

Now you can see why when a patient comes in and tells me about these symptoms I express pleasure rather than commiseration. Sometimes I warn them beforehand, but not always; that is a judgement I make at the time. Some people will be deterred from following the treatment if they know that things could get worse before they get better. Other people don't experience die-off at all, they simply start to improve and there would have been no need to tell them. However I always suggest they call in if they experience any change in their symptoms other than overall improvement. In a book, such as this, it is important to discuss the effect. If it occurs to you, continue with the treatment. If you are concerned, then it is time to consult a professional.

PART THREE
Meal Plans and Recipes

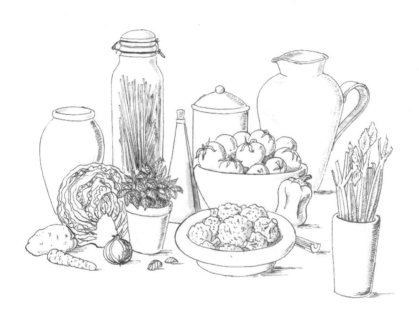

CHAPTER 8

Practical Suggestions

Now it's time to get down to the main purpose of this book: practical details of what you can eat while you are treating yourself. First, remind yourself of the 'Foods to Avoid at All costs' on pages 27–28. In the following meal plans and recipes these are avoided. However, some people with candidiasis can eat small amounts of fresh fruit, so some of the recipes do contain fruit, but few have fruit as a major component.

You will also come across mention of adjustments you can make depending upon whether your problem is mild or severe. If your symptoms are mild and you have only had the problem for a short while you may be able, for instance, to have the occasional piece of fruit, to risk the lactose in instant dandelion coffee or the possibility of moulds on herb teas. You may even be able to put a tiny amount of honey in a dessert. If the problem is severe, or if you have had it for a long time and it is proving difficult to beat, then you must be particularly strict with the diet and act accordingly. Obviously, if your problem is mild, but you are willing to accept the dietary restrictions and you want to get rid of it as fast as possible, then go on the strict version of the diet. This is a judgement you will have to make.

Detailed consideration has not been given to any other allergies and/or food intolerances you might have developed in addition to the candidiasis. That is beyond the scope of this book. If you react to specific foods then you will need to make the appropriate substitutes or consult an allergy cookbook; see my book *Living with Allergies* (Allen and Unwin, 1986).[1] However some thought has been given to allergy sufferers. For instance, many people are sensitive to milk; in addition it contains sugar (lactose) and may actually contribute to candida growth. You can make simple substitutions such as replacing cow's milk with unpasteurized sheep's or goat's milk, or milk substitutes made from rice, soya or oats. Similarly in recipes in which wheat flour is used you can use barley flour. In some of them you can even use a variety of other flours such as oatmeal flour or even chick pea or lentil flour. See for instance the recipes for making pastry (pages 75–6).

Most people's lives are already full. The simple chore of having to avoid certain foods and find specific substitutes takes some time. So where possible the suggestions below are aimed at keeping any extra time in the kitchen to a minimum.

POSITIVE ALTERNATIVES

If you are suffering from candidiasis you are almost certainly prone to leaky gut syndrome. In addition your immune system is already under stress. For both these reasons it is important to eat a diet with as few chemical additives as possible and to decrease the toxic load on your body. Thus the recipes are based as much as possible around natural foods rather than processed foods, and natural flavourings rather than artificial ones.

- Buy organically grown produce where possible to minimize your intake of toxins.
- Get your protein from fresh meat and fish, not smoked or processed, and, where possible, from free-range animals, reared organically.
- Include free-range eggs. Eggs make a quick and nutritious breakfast. As a result of the warnings about high cholesterol levels and heart attacks, eggs have suffered from a poor image for a while, because of their high cholesterol content. However, it's not the amount of cholesterol you eat that's important; it's the amount you make in your body. This depends largely on the amount of fat you eat and on the state of your liver. So keep

the fat content of your diet to a minimum and ensure you eat a diet that is rich in the B vitamins and in lecithin. Eggs are packed full of valuable nutrients, including the lecithin and B vitamins that you need. Be warned though, you should not eat the egg whites when they are raw, they must be cooked. Raw egg whites contain avidin, a substance that combines with biotin and prevents you absorbing it. Not only is biotin an essential nutrient for everyone, it is particularly important if you have candidiasis as it inhibits the metabolism of *Candida albicans* by keeping it in the non-invasive yeast form rather than in the invasive and more virulent mould form.

- Use lentils and dishes based on dried beans to increase your intake of filling foods since you can no longer eat bread.
- Use whole grains instead of refined grains. This is not only to get the extra nutrients, the vitamins and minerals, found in whole grains but lost in the milling and refining process, it's also because you will benefit from the additional fibre, which will improve the environment in your digestive tract and make life more difficult for the *Candida albicans*. There is a further benefit: because whole grains take longer to digest, to break down into individual glucose units, there is a slow, steady release of glucose molecules which can be absorbed rapidly, removing them from the gut where they could otherwise act as food for *Candida albicans*. When white flour or white rice is eaten the glucose molecules are released more rapidly; if this happens faster than their absorption and some remain in the gut to nourish and encourage the candida this is obviously not a desirable outcome.
- Eat generous helpings of fresh vegetables, both cooked and raw, in salads (using lemon juice instead of vinegar in the dressings).
- Unless you're trying to lose weight, eat raw seeds and nuts for snacks. Do not eat nuts or seeds that have been chopped or ground and stored; because of their high content of unsaturated fats they can go rancid very easily. Grind them as you need them.
- If you are looking for an alternative to butter, look for a margarine or spread that states clearly that it is non-hydrogenated. It is important that it is not hydrogenated as the

normal process of hydrogenating the vegetable oils results in toxic and unwanted compounds called trans-fatty acids.
- Use fresh herbs for seasoning (not dried as yeasts can collect on the leaves during the drying process), and ground spices.

WATER

Water is, or should be, a simple matter. Certainly there's rarely a problem with either yeasts or sugar when you drink water. However, normal tap water not only contains a variety of toxins, it often has an unpleasant taste, mainly due to the chlorine in it. In spite of all the purification, and in part as a result of it, there are many substances in tap water, from organic chemicals to toxic minerals, that can do you harm. This harm may be slight, the levels of toxins may be small, the water may have been passed as 'potable' (suitable for drinking), but over the long term, damage can result. While you are suffering from candidiasis it is particularly important to minimize the load of toxins your body has to deal with, in part because of the 'leaky gut syndrome' and in part because it already has so many to deal with from the candidiasis, both directly and indirectly.

For all these reasons you should plan to drink purified water or bottled water. Purified water you can make at home using either a 'reverse-osmosis' method or distillation. The equipment is available relatively cheaply, considering the benefit you will derive. A water filter is even cheaper, but it only removes a small proportion of the unwanted substances, and progressively removes smaller and smaller amounts of even these. Bottled water can be bought either sparkling or still. Still water is better than sparkling because of its lower phosphate level.

For the best of health you should use pure water, whether home purified or purchased, not only for drinking but for cooking as well. This means using purified water for boiling foods, such as pasta or rice, and for steaming vegetables. This improves the quality of what you cook since there are no toxins in the water for the food to absorb. It also means it is safe to use the water again or to drink it. Every time you cook food in water some nutrients are lost from the food and enter the water; by using this water you gain the benefit of these nutrients. Even when you steam vegetables some nutrients enter the water. You can store this water in the refrigerator and then use it to make sauces and gravy, especially if it is starchy water from cooking grains; you can use it to cook the next lot of vegetables, make it into a soup or drink it as it is. You may be surprised to find how much of the flavour is in the water.

USEFUL TIPS

Many people, particularly if they live on their own, are busy, or dislike cooking, fall into the habit of grabbing a quick snack when hunger strikes. This is often a sandwich, some biscuits or a quick takeaway meal such as a pizza. None of these foods are now permitted. Instead you may be faced with making a full meal – and decide you don't have the time, can't be bothered and the diet's too difficult. The following tips will help ease the situation and provide a suitable alternative.

- Pancakes (see pages 59–61) can be made in bulk and stored in the refrigerator between layers of grease-proof paper. Use instead of slices of bread.
- Brown rice can be cooked and then frozen. Freeze it in quantities suitable for individual servings. When you need it, boil some water in a pan and add the block of frozen rice. As soon as the rice is hot it can be served.
- Dried beans can be treated in the same way as brown rice. Choose haricot beans, lima beans, red kidney beans, or any other bean of your choice. Cook them, freeze them in individual serving-sized portions, then heat through when needed.
- Make it a habit, when cooking, to prepare double quantities. This usually takes only about 20 per cent more time. Serve half and deep freeze the other half, ready for a future meal.

Unlike other recipe books this section is full of eating ideas rather than just recipes. The focus has been given to the meal times and foods that are the most difficult when you are faced with the list of foods you cannot eat. Thus the emphasis is on breakfast ideas, snacks, lunches-on-the-run, biscuits and desserts; Chapter 12 shows how menu planning at home and menu selection when eating out allow you to keep to the treatment and still enjoy yourself.

1. *Living with Allergies* is available from the author.

CHAPTER 9

Breakfast

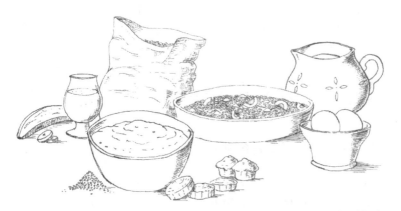

Breakfast is a particularly important meal, yet many people skip it or grab something on the run. Don't do this. For good health you need a good breakfast. The explanation is all to do with hormones.

Think back to times when we were nomadic or lived in caves. Food was not readily available, as it is now, from corner stores, late-night shops or deep-freezes. It took time, effort and luck to find food in the wild. The effort took energy, energy that had to come from the food you had previously eaten. It was important that this energy was used wisely, not squandered, and that if it was not needed it was stored as fat within the body. This is where the hormones come in. In the morning and during the daytime your hormones are (were) programmed to convert the food you eat into instant energy, so you can (could) go out and hunt with the best possible chance of success. To discourage you from sloth, and to preserve your stores of body fat for real emergencies, your body is (was) less keen to mobilize the stored fats and more inclined to stimulate your digestive juices. In the evening, when there is (was) little chance of you hunting successfully, your hormones are (were) programmed to convert your successfully garnered food, once eaten, into body fat.

When you have candida problems you are likely to be tired. By having a good breakfast you give yourself the best chance of increasing your energy during the day. This may not seem obvious at first, you may insist that you are not hungry in the morning, that you never have been. Yet much of this is habit, a habit that can be changed, and one that should be changed if you want to optimize your health and energy. In passing, it is worth pointing out, though you have probably recognized it already, that by eating a significant amount of your food in the morning rather than in the evening you are also likely to be slimmer.

PLANNING THE MEAL

One of the problems of a candida sufferer is that breakfast can be a particularly difficult meal to plan for. Standard breakfasts commonly include a variety of forbidden foods: fruit juice, dried fruit (in commercial muesli), fresh fruit (if your problem is severe), bacon, kippers, smoked meats, sausages, mushrooms, tinned tomatoes, slices of cheese, toast, croissants, marmalade, jam or sugar, whether on cereals or in tea or coffee. So some careful planning is necessary or you will find yourself, with only minutes to spare before you must rush off to work or get the children to school, gazing in dismay at kitchen cupboards that contain 'nothing you can eat' and with a brain running through the list of usual breakfasts and getting to the end before alighting on something you can prepare. You will then either go without and be reduced to looking for a snack of whatever you can get in the middle of the morning, and this too will probably contain sugar or bread, or else you may give up on the diet before you even start, telling yourself, in exoneration, it's all too hard.

Don't despair, there are many interesting breakfasts that you *can* make. You can have a variety of cereals and there are some interesting toppings you can have on them even though you must avoid sugar and possibly fruit. You can have a variety of hot dishes, even though you must avoid bacon and kippers, and you can use potato or rice instead of bread. Finally, you can do wonderful, quick and easy things with pancakes or scones, instead of toast, and yes, there are toppings you can put on them when once again you realize that you would normally be using something with a sugar base that must now be avoided.

The first thing to do is to prepare a mental list of several different menus that appeal to you and that you can have. Then plan the recipes, shop for the ingredients and have them ready to use. After that, the morning meal can become a question of selecting which of the many permitted meals you would like to have today. Here are some recipe ideas.

RECIPES

CEREAL DISHES

Be warned, the majority of brand-name cereals you buy in the supermarkets contain sugar, and not only small amounts; some are an amazing 50–60 per cent sugar. Since sugar is the perfect food for candida and you must avoid it, you will have to learn to identify these sugar-laden cereals and avoid them. Look for ones that carry the words 'sugar-free', and that do not list sugars (sucrose, glucose, frutose, lactose, maltose, manose) as ingredients. Notice that the names of most sugars end in -ose and use this as a guide.

Serve these cereals with milk (or substitute), or one of the flavoured milks described below, and learn to enjoy the flavour of the different cereals. In time you will wonder why you ever wanted to swamp them all in sugar.

With regard to milk, it's best to avoid pasteurized milk. Some people find it's best to avoid all cow's milk for several reasons, including the lactose (sugar) it contains, a possible intolerance and because, particularly when pasteurized, it can encourage candida. You will find milk substitutes useful. These include goat's and sheep's milk (if you are only sensitive to cow's milk) as these can often be bought raw. The sale of unpasteurized milk is illegal in some countries, and if this is the case where you live, or if your candida problem is severe, use milks made from soya, rice, oats or other plant foods, which can be bought in liquid form or as powders. In the following recipes the term 'milk' should be taken to include all these various forms of milk and its substitutes.

VANILLA MILK

milk powder or substitute such as soya milk powder
vanilla pods

Method
Keep three or four vanilla pods in a container of powdered skimmed milk (or substitute) and in time the powder will pick up the vanilla flavour. You can then blend this with water, with milk and water or with fresh milk to make a thickened, vanilla-flavoured milk.

If you have time you can place a vanilla pod in fresh milk or soya milk, bring to the boil and infuse off the heat until the milk has picked up the flavour, then serve this milk, hot or cold, within the next day or two. Keep the vanilla pod and use it again.

You could also use vanilla flavouring to achieve this effect but this is artificial, the pure pod is healthier.

NUTMEG, CINNAMON OR MACE MILK

1tsp/2tsp nutmeg, or cinnamon, or mace or a combination
50ml/3tbsp/¼C boiling water

Method
Add the boiling water to the spices, dissolve them and allow to cool then store in the refrigerator. Add a few drops of this liquid to the milk you are about to use.

Although not sweet in themselves these spices give an illusion of sweetness to the milk and make the final dish, the cereal and milk, more interesting.

SESAME MILK

You will be using tahini for this recipe. This is a paste made from ground sesame seeds, in the same way as peanut butter is a paste made from ground peanuts. You will be able to buy it from a health-food shop, some delicatessens, and shops specializing in Lebanese food.

Serves 1–2
50ml/3tbsp/¼C tahini
Fresh milk or substitute

Method
Put the tahini in a bowl and add the milk slowly, stirring thoroughly to blend. Initially the mixture will get thicker and thicker, then suddenly, as you add a little more milk, it will become quite thin.

Adjust the amounts of milk and tahini until you achieve a flavour that you like and use this instead of milk on cereals and desserts.

NUTTY MILK

nut butter
fresh milk or substitute

Method
Prepare this in the same way but use almond butter, cashew nut butter or some other nut butter instead of the tahini. Peanut butter should be avoided as peanuts often contain small amounts of mould (dead or alive).

OATMEAL PORRIDGE

Serves 1
50g/2oz/½C rolled or porridge oats
300ml/10fl oz/1¼C milk or water and water mixed
a pinch of salt (optional)

Method
If using raw rolled oats (as opposed to quick-cooking porridge oats), soak them in warm water overnight to reduce cooking time.

Combine the oats and the milk or water and heat gently until fully cooked. The amount of liquid used will depend on how thick or how runny you like the final porridge. You can adjust the amount during cooking. Salt can be added if desired.

Serve with a little milk or one of the milk substitutes.

Mixed Grain Porridge
Other grains can be used either in the form of rolled flakes, including wheat, barley, rye, corn, millet or rice, or in the form of meal or flour. They can be used individually or in combination.

Other Variations
Porridge can also be made with foods that are not grains, but are high in starch, such as buckwheat or cassava.

Many additions are possible for variety and interest. Nuts or seeds can be stirred in just before serving; try sunflower seeds, sesame seeds, pine kernels or chopped almonds, cashews or hazelnuts. Avoid peanuts or coconut. Toasted sunflower seeds or toasted almonds can be used as toppings. Spices such as nutmeg, mace or cinnamon can be added.

EGG DISHES

On a yeast-free diet eggs can be served in all the usual ways except that you cannot, of course, add cheese or mushrooms, and they cannot be served with toast. However they can all be served with pancakes, muffins (see pages 83–7), scones or rice cakes instead of the bread. Potatoes and rice also make a good balance to the richness of an egg dish.

POACHED EGGS ON MASHED POTATO

Serves 2
2 medium-sized potatoes, washed, peeled (if desired) and diced
2 eggs
milk
salt and freshly ground white pepper to taste

Method
Cook the potatoes in boiling water until soft. This should only take about 5 minutes. Meanwhile, poach the eggs in simmering water or in poaching pans over simmering water.

Strain and mash the potatoes, adding milk to the required consistency, and season.

Arrange a bed of mashed potatoes on a plate and place the two poached eggs on top. Serve.

SAUTÉED EGGS ON HASH BROWNS

Serves 2
1 onion, finely chopped
10ml/2tsp/2tsp olive oil
2 medium-sized potatoes, washed and grated
salt and freshly ground black pepper
2 eggs

Method
Sauté the onion in half the oil in a heavy-based frying pan until transparent then add the potatoes. Cook on a medium high heat, turning frequently, until tender. Season.

Move the hash browns to one side of the pan, add just enough of the remaining oil to the pan to prevent sticking, break in the eggs and cook gently until done to the required degree. The heat should not be so high that the bases of the eggs become browned, burnt or crisp.

Serve the eggs either on or beside the hash browns.

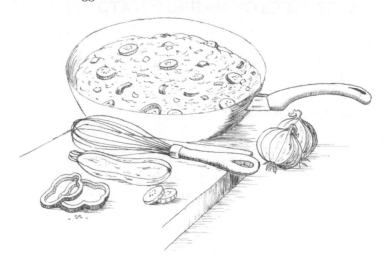

SPANISH OMELETTE

Serves 3
1 onion, finely chopped
1 green and 1 red pepper, (capsicum), finely chopped
10ml/1tbsp/1½tbsp olive oil
3–6 cooked potatoes (to balance the egg), diced
a few leftover vegetables if available
salt and freshly ground black pepper
6 eggs

Method
Sauté the onion and peppers in the oil until soft then add the potatoes and any other cooked vegetables and cook, covered, for 2–3 minutes. Season.

Beat the eggs lightly together and add the vegetables (reserving the oil), stirring carefully. Clean the pan, add half the reserved oil, and when hot the egg and vegetable mixture. When cooked on the base, remove the omelette, add the remaining oil, slide the omelette back into the pan, and cook the other side.

Serve flat, hot or cold.

LEFTOVERS

This is also the time to use your imagination and be adventurous. Have some non-traditional breakfasts. For example, you can eat food that's left over from the meal of the previous evening, such as:

Leftover casserole or stew served with pancakes.

Leftover mashed potato served with eggs, cooked any way you like.

Leftover pasta (spaghetti, macaroni, fettuccine, tagliatelle, etc.) incorporated into an omelette – make as for Spanish Omelette, using pasta instead of potato.

Leftover vegetables, chopped and used in Spanish Omelettes.

Leftover vegetables mixed in with pancake batter and made into fritters or pancakes.

Leftover rice, meat, chicken, fish or vegetables (or a combination) mixed together and lightly fried using a very small amount of oil.

BUBBLE AND SQUEAK

In Britain this dish is usually made with potato and cabbage, in New Zealand from carrot and pumpkin; it can be made with whatever combination of cooked vegetables you choose, or have available. If they are 'wet' it is helpful to use potato as well. Mash such vegetables as potato, parsnip or pumpkin, chop others finely.

Method
Combine the vegetables.

Lightly oil a frying pan and heat. Add the mixed vegetables and continue to heat. Turn frequently to avoid burning, but cook until the combination has browned.

Bubble, Squeak and Shout
Bubble and Squeak, but with added protein from fish, poultry or meat.

Method
Chop the meat or poultry, or flake the fish. Add to the hot lightly oiled, frying pan. Then add the various vegetables and cook as for Bubble and Squeak.

KEDGEREE

Kedgeree can be made from leftover rice and white fish with the addition of chopped hard-boiled eggs. For a main meal, poach the fish in water flavoured with parsley, bay leaf and lemon juice, then cook the rice in the poaching liquid.

Serves 1
olive oil
115g/4oz/1C cooked brown rice
55g/2oz/½C cooked white fish
1 hard-boiled egg, chopped
English mustard
salt and freshly ground black pepper

Method
Warm the olive oil in a skillet. Mix all the other ingredients together in a bowl. Add to the skillet, stir-fry gently until heated through, season and serve.

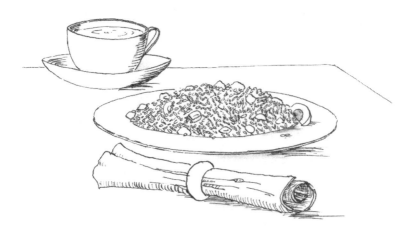

PANCAKES

Most people choose to make pancakes with self-raising flour and this is certainly the simplest way. However the baking powder added to plain flour to make it rise commonly contains aluminium to prevent it becoming lumpy, and aluminium is a toxic metal and not good for your health. There are two ways of getting around this. You can make your own baking powder using the recipe overleaf, or you can use beaten egg whites. The former is quick and easy to do, the latter takes a little longer, but makes tastier pancakes, and if you add extra eggs you can convert the pancakes into a protein-rich meal.

Pancakes can be made with other types of flour, particularly rye, oat or barley flour. Other types, such as buckwheat, soya or rice are generally less successful as they do not contain gluten. Use them for the small and stiffer pikelets. Adding an extra egg can improve their strength.

BAKING POWDER

2tsp/4tsp sodium bicarbonate
4tsp/8tsp cream of tartar

Method
Combine the ingredients, mix thoroughly and store in an air-tight jar. Use about 1tsp/2tsp of the mixture for 450g/1lb/4C of flour. If the mixture tends to be lumpy you can add an equal amount of corn flour. If you do this you will, of course, need to double the amount you use in the recipes.

PANCAKES

Makes 8–12 pancakes
140g/5oz/1¼C plain wholemeal flour
2 eggs, separated
250ml/8fl oz/1C milk (or substitute)
a little butter or oil (butter makes the better pancakes)

Method
Combine about three-quarters of the milk with the flour and add the egg yolks. Beat the egg whites until stiff and fold into the mixture. Add more milk, until the desired thickness is obtained – like thin cream.

Heat a skillet, add the butter or oil and pour in sufficient batter to nearly cover the base. Cook until bubbles form and the batter can be lifted from the pan. Turn, and cook on the other side. Lift out onto a plate. Repeat.

Sunflower Pancakes
Add sunflower seeds to the basic pancake batter. Cook as usual.

Pikelets
Use the basic pancake mixture but decrease the amount of liquid to make a firm mixture. Add a smaller amount of batter to the pan,

about one spoonful, such that it spreads out to about 5–7cm/2–3in in diameter. Several can be cooked in the pan at one time.

VEGETABLE FRITTER–PANCAKES

Pancake batter
Leftover vegetables

Method
Add the vegetables to the pancake batter, making sure there is enough batter to hold the fritters together.

Fry small amounts in a hot skillet until cooked and browned on both sides.

Storing Pancakes
Pancakes and pikelets can be made a day or two ahead of time and stored ready for use. Make them in the normal way. Place alternating pancakes and layers of greaseproof paper in a stack, wrap it in a tea towel and store in the refrigerator. Pikelets can be stored in an air-tight container.

They can then be treated much as you would a slice of bread, and made into 'sandwiches' or eaten in any of the ways described here for freshly cooked pancakes. If you have made them with additions to the batter they can be a ready-to-eat snack in themselves.

They can also be frozen. Thaw them at room temperature. Heat in the oven at 150°C/300°F/gas mark 2 or on a covered plate over a saucepan of boiling water.

Serving Suggestions
While the usual fillings are sweet, and therefore forbidden, there are several possible fillings or toppings that can be used.

If you can eat fresh fruit then add sliced or chopped fresh fruits.
Instead of cream, too fattening for daily use, make a thickened milk by adding skimmed milk powder to fresh milk. Add carob powder to give a chocolatelike flavour.

Use sesame milk or some of the nut milks, make these a little
thicker than usual (see page 53).

Use pancakes as a base for egg dishes, instead of toast.

Fill them with leftovers from the evening meal the night before.

SCONES

Makes 9–12 scones
200g/7oz/1¾C plain wholemeal flour
1tsp bicarbonate of soda
2tsp cream of tartar
a pinch of salt
50g/2oz/½ stick or 50ml/3tbsp/¼C butter or vegetable oil
150ml/5fl oz/⅔C fresh milk

Method

Sift together the flour, bicarbonate of soda, cream of tartar
and salt. Rub in the butter if using. Add the milk, and oil if using, and
mix lightly, handling it just sufficiently to create a homogeneous
dough. Roll out to a thickness of 2cm/1¾in. Use a pastry cutter or
small glass to create small circles. Place on a greased baking tray.

Bake in a preheated oven for 8–10 minutes at 220°C/425°F/
gas mark 7.

Optional: brush the scones with milk or beaten egg before
baking to create a 'glaze'. Note: you need the extra cream of tartar
as you are using fresh milk instead of soured milk.

Seed and Nut Scones

Add 50g/2oz/¼C sunflower seeds, sesame seeds or chopped nuts
to the basic recipe, after you rub in the butter/before you add the
milk.

Carob Scones

Replace 1tbsp/1½tbsp flour with 2tbsp/3tbsp carob powder.
Because carob powder is much sweeter than chocolate powder this

will (just!) give the illusion of being sweet, without the need for added sugar.

Muffins

The basic wholemeal muffin (pages 83–4) and the high-fibre chewy muffin (page 85) are ideal accompaniments to savoury meals.

Other Bread Alternatives

There are several other alternatives you can use to replace the bread that you cannot have – and remember, you cannot have any breads, even 'yeast-free' breads or soda bread.

Most health-food shops sell rice cakes. These are made from puffed brown rice, and are generally round. If you have tried them as they come in the packet and been unimpressed, try toasting them; you could be in for a pleasant surprise.

Some of the plain biscuits on the market, made from rye or whole wheat, say they are yeast free. Read the labels very carefully, however, and, if you are in any doubt at all, contact the manufacturer, preferably in writing so that you get a correct response, rather than the opinion of whoever answers the telephone. You do not want to find that after weeks, even months, of careful eating you have been unwittingly sabotaging your efforts by including a yeast-based biscuit in your diet.

DRINK YOUR BREAKFAST – BLENDED SHAKES

People in a hurry in the morning often choose to skip breakfast unless it can be made in under a minute. It is not a good idea to skip breakfasts, as we have already seen, so here are some very quick alternatives. All you need is a blender, a variety of appropriate ingredients and some imagination. Then it is simply a case of putting all the ingredients into the blender, hitting the switch for a few seconds, pouring out the result, preferably into an elegant glass (it can be washed up later), and drinking. If that still takes too long, pour it into a container with a lid, take it with you and drink when you do have time to sit down and relax, at least for a few minutes.

Remember that these blended breakfasts are 'foods' not 'drinks' and they should be consumed slowly, over a period of ten minutes or so, with a certain amount of 'chewing' so that there is time for the production of saliva and digestive enzymes. This may mean sipping at intervals while you are putting on your make-up, shaving or making the children's sandwiches. All this is far from ideal, of course, but I have found after over twenty years of advising people that this *is* what happens. The best I can do is to make suggestions so that what you eat is as nutritious as possible.

The liquid base

You can use unpasteurized cow's milk if available, and if you are not allergic or sensitive to it. Otherwise use unpasteurized goat's or sheep's milk, milk substitutes such as soya or rice milk, or diluted, unsweetened fruit juice if allowed. Do not use concentrated or sweetened fruit juices as a base as they will give you too much sugar. Instead of milk you can use cold fruit or herb teas such as rosehip or blended fruit teas, which give a pleasing flavour.

What you can add

There should be some protein. This can come from the milk or egg yolks; remember not to eat the raw whites. Soya milk powder (which is essentially cooked soya flour, or the dried version of soya milk) is a good protein source.

You can also add a variety of seeds, such as sunflower seeds, or nuts, such as almonds or Brazils. They do contain some protein but relatively little compared to their very high fat content, so use them sparingly. If you are using water or herb teas rather than milk as the liquid the ground nuts can add a pleasant richness to the drink. Do not use nuts or seeds that have been ground and then stored; because of their high unsaturated fat content they can go rancid very easily so always grind them as you need them. One way to do this is to place them in the blender first with a very small amount of liquid and blend until crushed, then add the other ingredients. You can also use tahini or pre-made nut butters (except peanut butter).

If you are constipated add linseeds, but if you do this you should drink the shake within five or ten minutes of making it otherwise it will 'thicken' and become glutinous as a result of the (beneficial) effect of the linseeds.

Chocolate tastes nice, but without the sugar usually added to it it's bitter. It is also in itself bad for you. Carob powder, on the other hand, is nutritious, pleasant tasting and very slightly sweet.

Dandelion coffee (available from health-food shops) is good for the liver and pleasant to taste. The 'instant' variety dissolves ready in a small amount of warm water.

If your candidiasis is mild and fruit has not been forbidden, you can add one piece of your chosen fruit to the shake.

SUNFLOWER SHAKE

Serves 1
1 glass of your chosen liquid
1 small banana
1 tbsp/2tbsp sunflower seeds

Method
Place the sunflower seeds in a blender, add sufficient milk to make a paste and blend. Add the rest of the milk and the banana. Blend until smooth and serve in a tall, elegant glass.

CAROB SHAKE

1 glass of your chosen liquid
2tsp/4tsp carob powder
a tiny pinch of nutmeg

Method
Blend all the ingredients and serve.

For speed, simplicity or if you don't have a blender, this can be made by shaking the ingredients together in a container with an air-tight lid.

HIGH-PROTEIN SHAKE

250ml/8fl oz/1C milk
1 egg yolk (remember not to eat the raw egg white)
1dsp/2dsp pine kernels
cinnamon to taste
sesame seeds and nutmeg to decorate

Method
Blend the milk, egg yolk, pine kernels and cinnamon until frothy. Decorate with a sprinkling of sesame seeds and a tiny sprinkle of nutmeg, and serve in a tall glass.

HIGH-FIBRE SHAKE

1 glass of your chosen liquid (dandelion coffee would be excellent, as it stimulates the liver)
1dsp/2dsp psyllium hulls
1 tsp/2tsp slippery elm
1dsp/2dsp linseeds
carob powder for flavouring

Method
Blend all the ingredients together. Drink immediately, as it will soon thicken.

CHAPTER 10

Snacks and Light Lunches

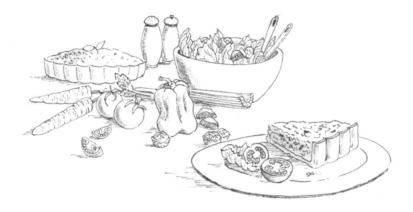

Finding a quick snack is often difficult, as the normally available snack foods commonly contain things that are forbidden. Sandwiches and snack foods that can be picked up near the workplace or on the road usually rely heavily on bread (yeast), burgers (yeast in the bun), salads with mayonnaise (vinegar), yoghurt and sugar. Crisps are not particularly healthy; some of them are over 50 per cent fat. A better bet is nuts, but many of the roasted nuts have been boiled in oil and that's not healthy either. So it's important that you plan and buy ahead: if you have a few pre-planned strategies you are less likely to be caught short and hungry with nothing you can eat. This chapter focuses on handy things to snack on at home or in the office, and on what you *can* buy when on the run. It also includes meals away from home. Main meal lunches, eaten at table, are covered in Chapter 12.

WHAT YOU CAN BUY

Raw nuts have several advantages. They are tasty, they are filling and satisfying, and they are convenient. You can put a bag of them in your handbag or briefcase and leave them there. When you're hungry they are immediately available. If you can eat fruit, an apple and a handful of almonds make a tasty and satisfying snack. You can nearly always find a vegetable shop where you can buy some tomatoes. Botanically they are definitely a fruit, so think of them as such and enjoy them. Their advantage is that they do not have as much sugar as the fruits we normally think of as fruit. You can also buy other vegetables, such as celery hearts, a sweet red capsicum (pepper), or a carrot.

In some health-food shops you can find unsweetened carob products, including unsweetened carob-coated rice cakes. Because carob is a lot less bitter than chocolate, it's pleasant to eat, even without added sugar.

For your lunch you may be able to buy a slice of quiche or open flan with a savoury filling. Obviously you must avoid ones that contain bacon, mushrooms, cheese or other forbidden food, but spinach or leek quiche, salmon or tuna quiche, and others, may well be free of forbidden foods. It's worth asking, but make sure you check up on *all* the ingredients, not just the main one(s).

Most salads available at salad and sandwich bars have a dressing on them that contains vinegar, but if you ask you may well be able to get an undressed salad, one made from ingredients that have no added vinegar. If you buy your lunch regularly from the same place you could ask them to prepare a salad specially for you.

PLANNING

In general, however, it's nearly impossible to be sure that you will be able to find what you want when you want it and so some pre-planning and forethought are essential, both for a lunch you can bring with you from home and for snacks you can keep in your bag or briefcase for an emergency. I know pre-planning can be a nuisance, but it is a necessary part of the treatment and if you don't do it your symptoms are likely to get worse, not better.

RECIPES

Since sandwiches feature so strongly in so many snacks and light lunches the following ideas are essentially sandwich alternatives.

Pancakes

We come again to the pancake, as we did at breakfast time (pages 59–62). Use the same basic pancake recipes, but make them a little stiffer and thicker so that they can be transported safely. Experiment for yourself, the following recipes are only ideas. As at breakfast, you could add seeds or ground nuts to the batter; or flavour it as below. Add tahini or other nut butters or any of the fillings below.

Once you set your mind to it you will find you can make an endless variety of pancakes, just keep in mind the filling you plan to use so that the flavours of the batter and of the filling blend well together – and only you can decide what you consider to be a successful blend.

You can use any filling you like, just as you would in a sandwich; however, softer fillings are usually more successful than hard ones. For example, if you're using chicken, rather than putting in a few large pieces of chicken it's better to chop the chicken into small pieces, so that when you roll the pancake they won't break through. If you want a salad filling then a coleslaw-type, with finely shredded vegetables, is more successful than one consisting of a few relatively large pieces of lettuce, tomato and cucumber. Just keep in mind that the dressing for the coleslaw must be made from lemon juice and not vinegar.

THE BATTER

For variety you can add flavourings to the pancake batter.

CURRY PANCAKES

One day, for instance, you might add curry powder (the amount will depend on your taste). If you like the flavour but not the heat, add generous amounts of powdered coriander, paprika or turmeric, or slightly lesser amounts of coriander, cumin or other spices. Experiment and find out what appeals to you.

HERB PANCAKES

You could also add a variety of herbs to the batter. For this it's best to use powdered herbs rather than the crumbled or fresh leaves. Avoid dried leaves because of mould. Basil powder, for instance, mixes well through the flour and makes a delicious batter to use with a tomato-based filling. Powdered sage, rosemary or thyme go well in pancakes to be wrapped round meat dishes, and add finely chopped chives or parsley to pancakes you plan to fill with salad ingredients or cooked vegetables. If you have the luxury of a home garden it's a simple matter to grow large amounts of these herbs. Even if you have only a small space, or a flat, you can grow them in tubs on the windowsills.

TABBOULEH PANCAKES

If you like tabbouleh but find it difficult to eat as a snack on the road, follow this suggestion. Pick a *large* handful of parsley (be generous), put it in a food processor and chop very finely. Add the liquid and flour (or pre-made batter if you already have some to hand) and make the pancakes as usual. Then fill this with a combination of chopped firm tomato and finely chopped white onions. Season with salt and freshly ground black pepper.

THE FILLING

Any type of cooked meat and fish can be used, including leftovers from dinner the night before, a curry for instance, or the remains of a stew or casserole, suitably drained. You can use cooked vegetables in a pancake; a substantial filling can be made by adding mashed potato to whatever meat or fish you choose, or combining it with other vegetables.

In this you have slightly more latitude than with sandwiches as bread goes soggy a lot more readily than pancakes do, so for pancakes the filling can be moister, in fact is often better if it is slightly moist.

Once you have chosen the filling, prepare the mixture in a bowl then spread it over the flat pancake. Roll the pancake firmly, lay it on a piece of greaseproof paper and roll this firmly round the pancake, twisting both ends securely.

Sandwiches can become misshapen if tossed into a bag containing other items. Pancakes are even more vulnerable, so use a lunch box to carry them.

CHICKEN PANCAKES

Makes 4 pancakes
100g/4oz/½C chicken, minced or finely chopped
50g/2oz/½C cooked, red and green peppers (capsicums), chopped
50g/2oz ¼C firm, ripe tomatoes, chopped
1tbsp/1½tbsp chopped chives

Method
Combine all the ingredients, fill the pancakes and roll them up.

EGG AND LENTIL PANCAKES

Makes 4 pancakes
85g/3oz/½C cooked brown or yellow lentils
4 hard-boiled eggs, finely chopped
1 stick celery, finely chopped
4tbsp/⅓C chopped chives or parsley
salt

Method
Combine all the ingredients, fill the pancakes and roll them up.

SALAD PANCAKES

Pancakes can be filled with salad or raw vegetables of almost any type. Just make sure that they are finely chopped so that the pancake can be rolled, and use a dressing to hold the ingredients together (make sure this is based on oil and lemon juice and not vinegar).

Coleslaw
Use finely chopped cabbage, grated carrot, grated apple, chives or finely chopped spring onion, greens (scallions) and caraway seeds.

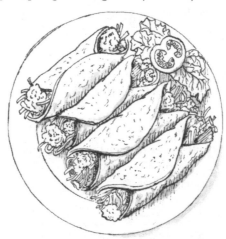

Combine these ingredients in your chosen proportions. Add mayonnaise or French dressing (made with lemon juice), just sufficient to moisten the salad without making it wet.

Spread over the pancake; add fish or meat if wanted.

Grated Parsnip
This may sound unusual, but is delicious. Grate a large parsnip, add some freshly squeezed lemon juice and mix thoroughly. When softened, spread this over the pancake. This is delicious on its own or with some flaked chicken added to it.

Grated Carrot and Orange Juice
Do the same thing with grated carrot and a small amount of freshly squeezed orange juice. Add chopped chives.

Nut and Seed Spreads
Peanut butter must be avoided because of the danger of it carrying the aflotoxin mould and the fact that peanuts are a relatively indigestible legume rather than a nut. True nuts are acceptable and you can use almond butter, cashew nut butter, hazelnut butter (but not the one with added chocolate!) and others. Tahini, the spread made by grinding sesame seeds, is also an excellent filler for pancakes.

They can be used on their own. They can also be combined with other ingredients and help to hold the other ingredients together.

PANCAKES PLUS SALAD

The pancake batter adds substance to the meal as well as holding the ingredients. If you add a salad you will add further nutritional value to the meal. This need not be anything elaborate, in fact it's better if it is not as salads can wilt. Instead, put large chunks of raw vegetables into a bag or box; a wedge of lettuce is usually more successful than torn leaves. Add half a carrot, a whole tomato, a large chunk of cucumber, half a pepper (capsicum), some radishes, etc. If you pack a small knife, preferably a folding one for safety, you can cut the vegetables into bite-sized pieces when you are ready to eat them.

Pastry-Based Snacks

Many people find pastry making difficult, especially with wholemeal flour. However, wholemeal flour is not only more healthy because of the fibre, vitamins and minerals it contains, but also because white flour delivers sugar (in the form of glucose) more rapidly than wholemeal flour and this can stimulate the candida. So in all the recipes below you are encouraged to use wholemeal flour and not refined white flour.

I was firmly in that category myself until, in self-defence, I evolved the following recipe. It came about by accident when I was determined, one Sunday evening when all the shops were closed, to have a final experiment with making pastry. Having got all the other ingredients together I found to my dismay and frustration that my cupboards contained no fat, apart from a few drops of olive oil, some French salad dressing and cream. Such was my determination and impatience I decided to experiment with this. As a dedicated non-pastry cook I was not sure of the difference between short pastry and, what, long pastry? However, it seemed to have something to do with the relative amounts of fat and liquid. I looked at some of the ratios, then I considered the cream. At about 30 per cent fat and 70 per cent water I figured the cream came somewhere in the range, so I simply added it to the flour and experimented. Here is the final recipe that resulted from that Sunday evening's trials. Since soon after that I was writing an allergy cookbook (*Living with Allergies*, available from the author), I also experimented with different types of flour. I found that you could use barley flour, oat flour or rye flour just as successfully. I then became more bold and tried with buckwheat, lentil, soya, rice, potato, chickpea and other flours. All of them worked. However, with the second group don't aim to lift the pastry off the rolling board intact. Instead, once you have rolled it out put the baking tin over the pastry; then tip all three, the board, the pastry and the baking tin, over, top to bottom, so the pastry can fall into the tin, and press it into place. Once cooked, however, even these unlikely pastries will produce a firm result that you can slice and take with you for a snack lunch. This is useful for people who are allergic or sensitive to the grains that contain gluten (wheat, barley, oats and rye). Exact quantities are not given in the recipes below because different flours absorb different amounts of liquid – you will find it's simple to get the consistency you want. If the mixture is too dry, add more cream; if it is too wet, add more flour.

Some patients' initial reaction to this recipe is that, being made with cream, this must be a very rich pastry. However, keep in mind the fact that butter is essentially the fat out of the cream, without the water, which you then add back in when making pastry the conventional way. Using cream means that the fat and water are already thoroughly mixed for you and this takes out the problem of having to recombine them. Do be sure to use fresh cream and not thickened cream that has had gelatine added to it.

If you're sensitive to dairy products, use the variation.

BASIC PASTRY

85g/3oz/¾C wholemeal flour
50ml/3tbsp/¼C cream that is approximately 30 per cent fat

These sample measurements allow for a thin pastry in a 20cm/9in flan dish. If you prefer a thicker pastry increase the quantities proportionately.

Method
Put the flour in a bowl. Add sufficient cream to make a smooth dough when worked lightly but thoroughly. Place on a board and roll out until thin, lift into a 9-inch pie tin or use in whatever other way you planned.

Not only is this easy to make, it also holds together well and does not need any special handling. As a further *big* advantage, it lifts cleanly out of the baking tin and so the washing up is easy.

Variation
20ml/1tbsp/1½tbsp vegetable oil
40ml/2tbsp/3tbsp water
85g/3oz/¾C wholemeal flour

These sample measurements allow for a thin pastry in a 20cm/9in flan dish. If you prefer a thicker pastry increase these quantities proportionately.

Method
Combine the vegetable oil with water in a ratio of 1 part of oil to 2 parts of water by volume. I keep a bottle of this in the fridge and it is ready for use any time I want it. Shake thoroughly and immediately add it to the flour, then work the two together thoroughly to form a soft and moist dough. If the resulting pastry is too wet, add more flour; if it is too dry, add more of the oil and water mixture. Allow it to 'rest' for 30 minutes if possible, as it then rolls out more easily. However this is not essential. Form the mixture into a ball with your hands. Sprinkle a little flour on the board, place the dough on it, knead lightly once or twice, and roll out the pastry.

You will find, as you adjust the quantities and practice, that, provided you have shaken the oil and water together thoroughly immediately before use, you can make a very thin pastry this way, with little trouble, that handles easily.

If you add a few teaspoons of lecithin granules to the oil and water mixture and shake the three ingredients together you will find that the oil and water do not separate afterwards, and the pastry is even easier to make.

This pastry can be used for making pies and tarts. Use it for quiches, flans and pasties, so you have a quick and simple lunch. It is also used in such recipes as Pear Dumplings (page 214) and as a basis for biscuits.

QUICHE

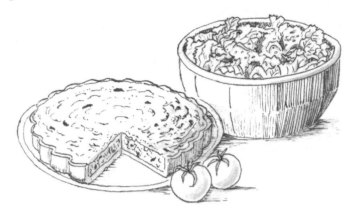

There are many different fillings you can put into a quiche, and some examples are given below. However, you can go far beyond some of the normal quiche recipes, and you can create several fillings that contain very few eggs, or even omit them altogether if you want to keep your egg intake down. You can also omit the cream if you want to reduce your fat intake or are sensitive to dairy products. For all the recipes below, use the Basic Pastry recipe or the variation, roll it out, line a 20cm/9in lightly oiled flan dish or baking tin.

SALMON QUICHE

Serves 2–4

1 pastry case, made with 85g/3oz/¾C wholemeal flour, part baked
200g/7oz salmon, either cooked or tinned
3 eggs, beaten
200ml/7fl oz/1C single/light cream
salt and freshly ground black pepper

Method
Make pastry, as previously described. Roll out the pastry and line an oiled baking tin.

Flake the salmon. Add the eggs and mix well, pour in the cream, season, mix and pour into the part-baked pastry shell. Bake at 180°C/350°F/gas mark 4 for 40 minutes.

Serve with a generous serving of sliced cucumber tossed in French dressing made with lemon juice.

SPINACH QUICHE

Serves 2–4
1 pastry case, made with 85g/3oz/¾C wholemeal flour
550g/1¼lb spinach, cooked, and very well drained
3 eggs, beaten
200ml/7fl oz/scant 1C single/light cream
nutmeg (freshly grated if possible)
salt and freshly ground black pepper
2tbsp/2½tbsp pine kernels

Method
Combine the spinach, eggs and cream. Season and sprinkle the pine kernels over and press in lightly. Bake at the same temperature for 40 minutes.

COCK-A-LEEKIE QUICHE

Serves 2–4
1 pastry case, made with 185g/3oz/¾C wholemeal flour
50g/2oz/¼C butter
200ml/7fl oz/1C milk
1 large potato, cooked and peeled
2 large or 3 small leeks, quartered, cooked and drained well
3 eggs, beaten
salt and freshly ground black pepper

Method
Use the butter and milk to mash the potato (it will be very moist), and combine with the leeks and eggs. Season and fill the pastry shell. Bake at the same temperature for 40 minutes.

QUICHE WITH LEFTOVERS

If you think that making a quiche, either for eating at home or for taking to work as a packed lunch, is too time consuming, use this idea. Cook double quantities of whatever you are having for dinner. During the last few minutes while you are waiting for it to cook you will have time to whip up the pastry, roll it out and line a buttered or oiled baking tin with it. Put the oven on to preheat, if it is not already being used to cook the dinner. Break as many eggs as you are going to use into a bowl and stir.

When you have dished up the meal, put the extra food into a bowl, flake or cut it into small pieces, pour over the eggs, mix quickly so as not to 'cook' the eggs, use some liquid from the cooking to achieve a moist consistency and turn the mixture into the pastry shell and pop the lot into the oven. With practice you will find you can do this so fast it can be cooking while you are eating.

It may well be cooked by the time you are ready to do the washing up and you can do the lot at once. Put the quiche into the refrigerator and it is ready for lunch the next day. If you plan carefully you can even make more than one and this should give you lunch and snacks for two or three days.

Quiches Without Egg

You may be concerned about the amount of eggs you are eating, especially if you are already having them for breakfast. It is very simple to make a 'quiche' or savoury flan, without using eggs at all. Simply follow the suggestions for Quiche With Leftovers but omit the eggs. To ensure the ingredients hold together add a handful of rolled oats and moisten with stock, milk or water, as available. Alternatively you can replace the rolled oats with rice or mashed potato.

CHAPTER 11

Afternoon Tea

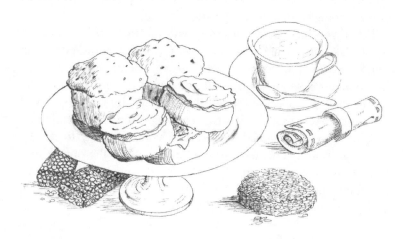

PLANNING THE MEAL

This can be an important meal socially, particularly for women who are not working, for older people, for people at clubs and so on. It is also hazardous if you have candidiasis as it is usually based round bread, sugar, dried fruit and other forbidden foods.

Some people, faced with their food restrictions, will choose to forgo the meal entirely. They may even choose to forgo the occasion – the card game, the game of bowls, or other activity. This is a mistake as you are now into double deprivation, the food and the occasion, and this can lead to loneliness, breaking the diet, or both. Don't do it.

If you are going out for afternoon tea and are unsure of what you will be able to eat when you get there (possibly nothing!), then take your own. That will involve a certain amount of effort and planning on your part but no one said that sticking to this diet was easy or without some inconvenience. The aim is to reduce the difficulty as far as possible. If you are the host(ess) there is less of a problem, you can ensure that at least some of the food you provide is appropriate for your own needs.

RECIPES

BREAD-SUBSTITUTE SANDWICHES

Although you can't use bread, if you use your imagination you can make yourself 'sandwiches' using other materials for support instead. These can include many of the plain and unsweetened biscuits made from rye or wholemeal wheat flour, pikelets (see pages 60–1), or rice cakes (bought in your local health-food store). Use exactly the same fillings as you would in bread-based sandwiches.

Scones (see pages 62–3) are also an excellent alternative; serve them simply with butter. If you're sensitive to butter use a substitute, such as olive oil spread, or liquid olive oil; fresh avocado is delicious, so is tahini. You can also use a non-hydrogenated soya margarine.

CAKES

Cakes are generally sweet, there's no getting away from that. They nearly all contain sugar or honey. If not, they are usually laden with fruit, either fresh or dried, or fruit juice. In the recipes below these ingredients have been omitted. If you are able to cheat a little, if you can add a small amount of sugar or honey to your diet, then do so. However, if you can't the recipes are still tasty. I won't claim that they are as mouth-wateringly delicious as cakes made with lashings of sugar and cream (if you like that sort of thing), but if you feel in the need of something close to cake then I've been assured over the years by desperate patients that these are a lot better than nothing!

HIGH-PROTEIN NUT CAKE

This one is truly delicious, even without sugar, if you enjoy nuts.

8 eggs
500g/18oz/4C ground nuts (choose from walnuts, almonds, cashews, etc. either singly or in combinations, but not peanuts)
1 tbsp honey (if permitted)

Method
Separate the eggs. Mix the yolks with the nuts and (if permitted) honey. At this point the mixture will only be partially wet.

Beat the egg whites until stiff. Add approximately a quarter of the beaten egg whites to the nut mixture and stir in. At this stage the mixture is so dry it is difficult to fold them in. Add another quarter of the beaten egg whites, this time folding them in. Repeat until all the egg whites have been folded in, trying to keep as much air in the mixture as possible. Place in a lightly buttered cake tin and bake at 160°C/325°F/gas mark 3 until the knife comes out clean.

Alternatively, drop spoonfuls of the mixture onto an oiled baking tray and make individual small cakes.

This is a high-protein cake and can be used as a snack if you 'don't have time for a meal'. It can also be served in combination with a first course that is mainly rice or pasta and vegetables, with very little protein.

Since it's slightly dry, serve with Vanilla Cream (page 129) or one of the Nutty Milks (page 53).

POPPY SEED POTATO CAKES

500g/18oz potatoes, cooked, cooking water reserved
40g/1¼oz butter or 1tbsp/1½tbsp vegetable oil
75g/2½oz/⅓C wholemeal flour
75ml/4tbsp/⅓C poppy seeds
vanilla essence

Method

Mash the potatoes until smooth with three-quarters of the butter or vegetable oil. Sprinkle the flour over the potatoes and mix in. Add a small amount of the hot potato water, just sufficient to ensure the flour is moist and well mixed in. Mix in the poppy seeds and add a few drops of vanilla essence to taste. Shape into small balls, place on an oiled baking tray and flatten. Bake in a preheated oven at 180°C/350°F/gas mark 4 for 45–60 minutes until lightly browned (the more water you add the longer it will take).

As a variation, replace the vanilla with 2½tsp/3tsp ground ginger. This is a lot of ginger but it helps to make up for the lack of sugar.

BASIC WHOLEMEAL MUFFINS

Traditionally these are made with a small amount of sugar, but you can omit the sugar and still enjoy the muffin. Try the following basic recipe and then experiment with variations of your own.

Makes 10–12 muffins
225g/8oz/2C wholemeal, barley or oat flour
1½tsp/2tsp Baking Powder (page 60)
2 eggs
250ml/8fl oz/1C milk
3tbsp/¼C vegetable oil

Method

Mix together the flour and baking powder. Beat the eggs and combine with the milk and oil. Add the dry ingredients. Place portions in a well-oiled muffin tray and bake at 180°C/350°F/gas mark 4 for about 15 minutes. (Larger muffins will take longer.)

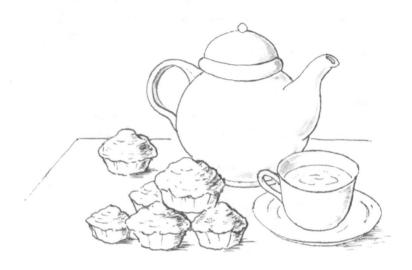

SPICED MUFFINS

For variety add different spices to the muffin mixture.

VANILLA MUFFINS

Add vanilla essence to the basic mixture; the amount will depend on your taste.

NUT AND SEED MUFFINS

Add 25g/1oz/¼C of poppy seeds to the basic recipe, or add toasted sunflower or sesame seeds. You can also add a variety of chopped nuts.

TAHINI MUFFINS

Replace the oil with twice the amount of tahini and reduce the amount of milk slightly. The exact proportions will depend on the amount of oil in the tahini you use. Since, when standing, the oil comes to the top of the tahini, you may find that by the bottom of the jar the tahini is much drier than at the top. Adjust the amount of milk you use accordingly, or add a little more oil if necessary.

SPICY FRUIT MUFFINS

This is another way to create the illusion of sweetness. Use mixed spice and grated orange and lemon rind – they should be organic as you do not want the chemicals that are put on the skin. The amounts of spice and rind are up to you and your taste buds. Sample small amounts of the dough, but remember the taste will be a little stronger when they are cooked. Add the spice to the flour and other dry ingredients, and the finely grated rind to the egg and milk mixture, then proceed as for the basic recipe.

HIGH-FIBRE CHEWY MUFFINS

If you want to add fibre to your diet substitute bran for some of the flour. You could also add some wheat germ; this is lower in fibre than the bran but adds a pleasing flavour. The more flour you replace the less milk you will need and the chewier will be the muffins. The result may be more like a bread and be appropriate to have with savoury meals.

BANANA MUFFINS

These muffins use only one banana, and working on the assumption that it is more starch than sugar you may find this an acceptable cheat.

Makes 6–10 muffins
1 egg
1 banana (*just* soft enough to mash, not soft enough to be too
   sugary and sweet)
1 tbsp/1½tbsp vegetable oil
a small pinch of salt
1 tsp/1 tsp Baking Powder (page 60)
115g/4oz/1C wholemeal flour
65ml/3½tbsp/¼C milk

Method

Beat the egg and mash in the banana, add the oil and mix. Sprinkle
the salt and baking powder over the flour and stir well. Add this,
gradually, to the egg and banana mixture, finally adding the milk.

Place portions into well-oiled muffin tins and bake in a preheated
oven at 180°C/350°F/gas mark 4 for 15 minutes or until well
cooked. Test with a sharp knife which should come out clean.

SOYA BEAN AND CAROB MUFFINS

If you can't have the banana in the Banana Muffin recipe, then
these muffins may be the ones for you.

Makes 10–12 muffins
2 eggs
150ml/5fl oz/⅔C milk
1 tbsp/1½tbsp vegetable oil
115g/4oz/1C wholemeal flour
115g/4oz/1C soya flour
55g/2oz/½C carob flour
2tsp/2tsp Baking Powder (page 60)
a pinch of salt

Method

Beat the eggs and combine with the milk and oil. Combine the dry
ingredients and mix well, then add them to the egg and milk. Mix
thoroughly. Adjust the amount of milk so you have a moist but firm

dough. Form into individual muffins. Place them in a well-oiled muffin tin and bake in a preheated oven at 180°C/350°F/gas mark 4 for about 15 minutes or until well baked.

BISCUITS

Most biscuits are sweet, so the same comments apply to biscuits as apply to cakes. However the lack of sugar does seem slightly less of a problem with biscuits. An example of this is this almond shortbread.

POPPY SEED FLAPJACKS

Makes 18–24 flapjacks
250g/9oz/3C rolled oats
120g/4oz/½C butter, melted
25g/1oz poppy seeds
20ml/1tbsp/1½tbsp honey (if permitted)

Method
Combine the rolled oats, butter and poppy seeds. Add honey (if permitted) or a small amount of boiling water, just sufficient to make a very lightly moistened mixture. Press into shallow oiled biscuit trays and bake in a preheated oven at 190°C/375°F/gas mark 5 for 30 minutes. Cut into squares while warm, then allow to cool. Remove the flapjacks from the tray and store in an airtight container.

SIMPLE BISCUITS

Basic pastry variation (page 76)
Spices, seeds, nuts, as desired

Method
Make the pastry and then experiment with flavours and additions.
　　Add a variety of spices such as cinnamon, nutmeg, allspice, mace or ginger. You can even add cumin or coriander for a semi-savoury taste.

Add ground nuts, such as ground almonds or ground walnuts.

Add seeds such as sesame seeds or sunflower seeds.

You may need to add slightly more of the cream to accommodate the added ingredients. Roll the mixture flat, keeping it biscuit-thick, rather than pastry-thin. Cut into squares and bake at 180°C/350°F/gas mark 4 until lightly browned. Alternatively simply spread it out on an oiled baking tray, run a sharp knife along it to divide it into squares, and bake at the same temperature.

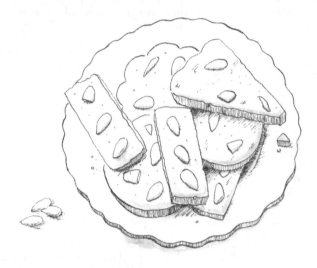

ALMOND SHORTBREAD

Makes 6–8 biscuits
200g/7oz/1½C flour
50g/2oz/⅓C ground almonds
125g/4½oz/½C butter
2 eggs
1tsp/1tsp almond essence
slivered almonds to decorate

Method

Mix the flour and almonds and rub in the butter. Break the eggs into a bowl and beat with a fork until the whites and yolks are well mixed; stir in the almond essence. Add the eggs to the flour mixture and mix well to form a stiff dough.

Roll out flat, cut into shapes and decorate each biscuit with the slivered almonds. Alternatively, spread the mixture over a baking tray, mark into squares with a sharp knife, and then decorate with the slivered almonds. Bake in a preheated oven at 180°C/350°F/ gas mark 4 until lightly browned.

CHAPTER 12

Main Meals

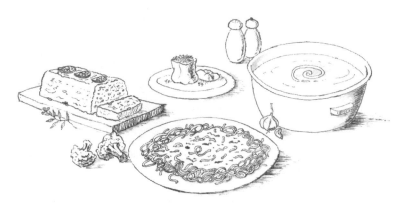

In this section we will be covering the main meal of the day, either lunch or dinner. Planning starts, as always, with shopping. Make sure your kitchen has a wide range of the foods you are allowed to eat.

On the whole vegetable dishes present few problems, as we shall see. Even main dishes are not too much of a problem. Most recipe books have a large number that you will be able to eat, either as they are described or with minor alterations. You may, for instance, have to eliminate the mushrooms from the recipe, substitute freshly cooked and drained tomatoes for tomato paste, or use chilli powder rather than, say, a sweet chilli sauce. A cheese sauce can be replaced by a parsley sauce or a sauce containing chives or other fresh herbs. Breadcrumbs, used to give a crusty topping, can be replaced by sesame seeds. For this reason only a few recipes are given here and this is a relatively small section.

STARTERS

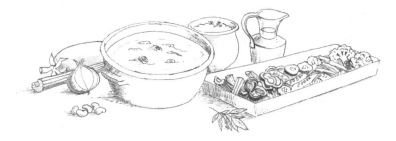

SOUPS

Soups make an excellent start to a meal, either hearty, such as the potato soup or borsch, or light, such as the chicken consommé or its variations, and should present few problems. However, you must avoid most stock cubes as they frequently contain yeast extracts.

POTATO SOUP

Serves 6
500g/1lb/1lb potatoes, peeled and diced
1 medium onion, chopped finely
900ml/1²/₃pts/4C soya milk
30g/1oz/2tbsp butter or 1¹/₂tbsp/2tbsp olive oil
1tbsp/1¹/₂tbsp barley flour
salt and freshly ground black pepper
a small bunch of watercress

Method
Place the potatoes and the onion in a saucepan of water and bring to the boil, then cover and simmer for about 30 minutes or until cooked. Drain. Add the soya milk and heat until simmering again.

Heat the butter or oil in a skillet, add the flour and cook until lightly browned, add to the soup and stir until thickened. Liquidize if desired.

Season and serve, decorated with watercress.

BORSCH

Traditionally, this is made with beef. In Britain, where it is no longer legal to sell beef bones, use lamb.

Serves 4
300g/10oz meat with stock bones
1kg/2¼lb beetroot
1 bay leaf
1 large onion, chopped
1 small celery stalk, chopped
1 carrot, grated
200g/7oz red cabbage, shredded
1tbsp/1½tbsp fresh lemon juice
salt and freshly ground black pepper

Method
Boil the meat and bones in 2 litres/3½pts/9C of water until thoroughly tender. Remove the meat, discard the bones, strain into a china dish, cool completely and remove the fat. Meanwhile boil the beetroot, cool and peel.

Add the bay leaf, onion, celery, carrot and red cabbage to the stock and bring to the boil. Add the lemon juice and simmer for 15 minutes. Slice the meat and grate the beetroot and add both to the soup.

Blend in a food processor, if desired; serve with a swirl of fresh cream.

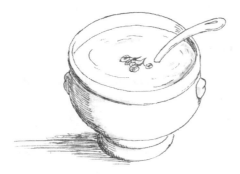

CHICKEN CONSOMMÉ

Serves 2
bones from 1 chicken
1 medium onion, chopped
1 small celery stalk, chopped
1 carrot, sliced
2 bay leaves
1 egg white
100g/3½oz chicken, minced or very finely chopped
salt and freshly ground black pepper

Method
Bring the chicken bones, vegetables and bay leaves to the boil in
1 litre/1¾pts/4½C of water and simmer for 1 hour. Allow to cool
completely and remove the fat.

Beat the egg white through the stock and then strain. Add the
minced chicken to the strained stock, simmer for an hour, adding
more water if it becomes too concentrated. Strain, season and serve.

Variations
Other meats can be used instead of chicken; it is delicious with
pork, or you can use fish and a fish stock instead.

Slice a variety of vegetables into fine strips and add to the soup
for the last 10 minutes.

ANTIPASTI AND DIPS

ANTIPASTI

Antipasti are a challenge, since normally many of the vegetables are pickled and the marinade normally contains vinegar. However, you can work with lemon juice for a refreshing change. Remember to use fresh herbs, not dried. Do not leave the vegetables to soak for long in the marinade or some fermentation may occur.

DRESSING:
juice of 1 lemon
1 clove garlic, crushed
1tsp/1½tsp each of fresh oregano, fresh parsley, fresh basil and fresh dill
1 pinch each of caraway seeds and cumin seeds
4tbsp/⅓C virgin olive oil

Method
Simmer all ingredients except the oil for five minutes. Cool, pour into a jar and add the olive oil.

VEGETABLES:
Cut a variety of vegetables into bite-sizes pieces or strips. The following suggestions are simply a guideline: small florets of cauliflower and broccoli, sweet peppers (capsicums) in all colours, green beans, mini-corns, celery, zucchini or courgettes and carrots, lettuce leaves
walnuts, almonds

Method
Shake the jar containing the dressing and pour over the vegetables in a bowl. Allow to stand for an hour, stirring frequently. Place lettuce leaves on a flat serving plate and arrange the vegetables. Serve garnished with fresh herbs and raw walnuts and almonds.

BROAD BEAN DIP

Serves 4

200g/7oz/1C dried broad beans, soaked in water overnight and
    drained
2 onions, chopped
100ml/4fl oz/¼pt olive oil
juice of 1 lemon
fresh herbs such as parsley, basil, chives, chervil – finely chopped
salt and white pepper

Method

Cover the onions and beans with water and boil until the beans are
completely soft. Drain, push the beans and onions through a fine
sieve, discarding any residue (if you're feeling lazy you can simply
blend them in a food processor), then add the oil and the lemon
juice and mix thoroughly. Add the herbs and season.

Serve with vegetable crudités.

HUMMUS

450g/1lb/3C dried chick peas
¼tsp/½tsp bicarbonate of soda
2 large cloves garlic (to taste)
juice of 1 lemon (to taste)
250ml/8fl oz/1C tahini
    (stir before using)
olive oil
paprika
cumin
parsley

Method

Cover the chick peas with cold water to which you have added the
bicarbonate of soda and soak overnight.

Drain off this water, add more water to cover and bring slowly to the boil; simmer, removing the froth as it comes to the surface, and making sure the peas remain totally covered by water. Cook for about 1½–2 hours, or until a pea can be completely crushed between two fingers, with no hard part in the middle. Drain and reserve the cooking liquid.

Allow to cool, liquidize using as much of the cooking liquid as is needed to achieve the desired degree of thickness. (This can be frozen and used as needed.)

Pulverize the garlic and add, with the lemon juice and tahini. The end result can be as runny or as thick as you choose, depending on the amount of liquid used.

Decorate with olive oil and powdered paprika, ground cumin and sprigs of parsley.

Serve with vegetable crudités.

MAIN COURSE DISHES

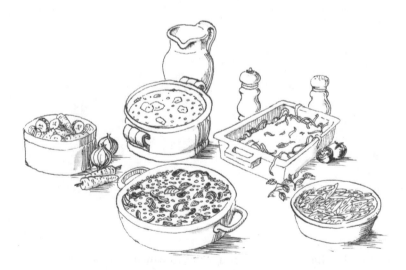

POACHED SALMON AND CUCUMBER WITH DILL

Serves 4
4 salmon steaks
5 sprigs of fresh dill
1 cucumber
1 lemon, halved
salt

Method
Slice the cucumber very thin, lay the slices on a flat plate and sprinkle salt liberally over them. Leave for at least an hour, several hours if possible.

In a flat pan place the salmon steaks and just sufficient water to cover them. Add the dill and the juice of one lemon half and simmer very gently until the salmon separates readily from the bone, about 6–10 minutes.

Drain the cucumber thoroughly, arrange on each plate, drain the salmon, and place the steaks on top of the cucumber. Garnish with slices of lemon and fresh sprigs of dill.

Serve with cooked vegetables such as carrots or peas, and potato.

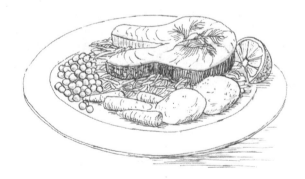

BAKED FISH

Serves 4

900g/2lb filleted lemon sole, plaice or similar fish – make sure the skin has been removed from both sides and choose 4 thick, substantial fillets, not small ones that break up
4 tomatoes
1 onion, minced
green tops of several shallots, 2cm/³⁄₄in long
15g/¹⁄₂oz/1tbsp butter
salt and freshly ground black pepper
500ml/16fl oz/1pt fish stock, made from the head, tail and bones
4 small sprigs of parsley

Method

Fold each fillet in three with the smooth side inside and place in a lightly buttered or oiled baking dish with the middle section uppermost.

Nick the tomatoes' skins, place in boiling water for about 60 seconds or until the skin can be removed easily. Remove the skin, scoop out the centres and discard and mash the flesh. Put the mashed flesh over the fish.

Sauté the onion and green shallot tops in the butter and pour over the fish. Season. Add just sufficient stock to prevent drying and to provide a small amount of sauce (add more during cooking if necessary) and bake for about 20 minutes at 180°C/350°F/gas mark 4. Decorate with the parsley; spoon the sauce around.

Serve with mashed potato and steamed vegetables (peas are excellent).

CURRIED PORK WITH LENTILS

Serves 4
20ml/1tbsp/1½tbsp olive oil
3 cloves garlic, crushed
2 medium or 1 very large onion, chopped
3tsp/6tsp ground coriander
2tsp/4tsp ground turmeric
1tsp/2tsp ground cumin
¼tsp/½tsp ground fenugreek
¼tsp/½tsp ground cardamom
¼tsp/½tsp ground allspice
1tsp/2tsp hot chilli powder (use more or less to taste)
400–675g/1–1½lb pork fillet or tenderloin, cut into bite-sized
  pieces
115g/4oz/1C red lentils
575–850ml/1–1½pt/2½–4C vegetable stock
2 carrots, chopped
2 potatoes, diced
2 green pepper (capsicums), diced

Method

Heat the oil in a wok or large-based skillet, add the garlic and the onion and toss for a minute. Combine all the spices, then add to the pan and stir until the onions and garlic are coated in them.

Add the pork fillet, toss until covered in spices, stir and cook for a few minutes until the surfaces of the meat are sealed.

Add the lentils and again stir until thoroughly mixed. At this stage you must keep stirring as the mixture is very dry.

Add stock to cover and simmer until the pork is nearly cooked, then add the vegetables (with more stock if necessary) and cook until tender. Serve with brown rice.

LAMB SHISH KEBAB

Serves 4
1kg/2¼lb lamb flesh, cut into bite-sized pieces
2 large green peppers (capsicums)
2 large red peppers (capsicums)
2 onions
several cherry tomatoes
marinade:
1 large onion, finely chopped
20ml/1tbsp/1½tbsp olive oil
40ml/2tbsp/3tbsp fresh lemon juice
a generous sprig of fresh rosemary (or other herb, to taste), chopped
salt and freshly ground black pepper

Method
Combine the marinade ingredients and stir in the lamb. Allow to marinate for several hours, or overnight, stirring occasionally, then remove the meat from the marinade and drain.

Thread the meat onto skewers, alternating it with chunks of the peppers, slices of onion and the cherry tomatoes.

Grill the kebabs under a hot grill, turning occasionally, until the lamb is cooked and the vegetables are browned. This should take 10–20 minutes depending on the size of the pieces and whether you like rare or well-cooked meat.

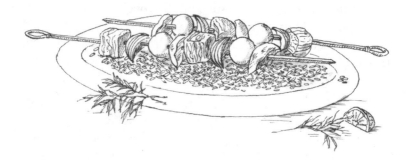

TARRAGON CHICKEN WITH JULIENNE OF VEGETABLES

Serves 4
30ml/1½tbsp/2tbsp olive oil
2 cloves garlic, crushed
2 onions, finely chopped
2 leeks, finely chopped
4 chicken quarters
2 large sprigs fresh tarragon
575ml/1pt/2½C chicken stock
225g/8oz/1C brown rice
very thin slices of 2 carrots, 2 peppers (capsicums), 2 stalks of celery,
    4 shallots, etc.

Method

Heat the olive oil and sauté the garlic, onions and leeks for 3 minutes. Add the chicken and sauté until sealed (add a touch more olive oil if necessary to prevent sticking) then add the tarragon and sufficient stock to cover the chicken. Cover and simmer until the chicken is tender (about 35–40 minutes). Meanwhile, cook the rice. Set the chicken aside, with the tarragon, keep warm, and reduce the liquid until it is a rich gravy (do not thicken).

To serve: make a ring of the rice. Fill the centre with the julienne of vegetables. Place the chicken pieces and tarragon on top and pour the concentrated sauce over the chicken.

CHICKEN OR PORK CASSEROLE

Serves 4
50ml/3tbsp/¼C olive oil
3 cloves garlic, crushed
3 onions, sliced into rings
1 green, 1 red and 1 orange pepper (capsicum), sliced into rings
4 tomatoes, sliced into rings
2 leeks, sliced
4 chicken legs or 450g/1lb pork fillet tenderloin
50ml/3tbsp/¼C brandy
575ml/1pt/2½C chicken or vegetable stock
1 sprig fresh marjoram

Method
Heat the olive oil in a pan and lightly sauté all the vegetables, then place them in casserole dish, reserving the oil. Sear the chicken or pork in the pan until lightly browned and lay on top of the vegetables. Add the brandy and marjoram to the pan and heat, then pour the whole contents of the pan over the meat. Bring the stock to the boil, and add just sufficient to cover the bottom of the pan and make a small amount of gravy. Cook in a preheated oven at 180°C/350°F/gas mark 4 for 1½ hours, adding more stock if necessary.

Serve with mashed potatoes and steamed vegetables.

BAKED EGGS

30g/1oz/2tbsp butter or 2tbsp/2½tbsp oil or substitute
2 large white onions, sliced
1 clove garlic, chopped
1 green pepper (capsicum), sliced in very thin rings
3tbsp/¼C freshly squeezed lemon juice
salt and freshly ground black pepper
450g/1lb/2C mashed potato
3 tomatoes, sliced
6 eggs
sesame seeds

Method
Heat the butter or alternative and sauté the onions and garlic until lightly coloured, then add the pepper. When cooked, add the lemon juice and season.

Oil a baking dish and spread the mashed potato round the edge. Fill the centre with the onion and pepper mixture, arrange the tomatoes on it, then break the eggs gently and place them evenly over the tomatoes. Sprinkle the sesame seeds over the top, and bake in a preheated oven at 180°C/350°F/gas mark 4 until the eggs are cooked.

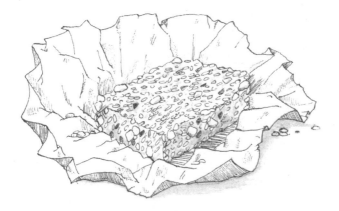

NUT LOAF

This makes an excellent main course dish. It can also be eaten cold, so take a slice to work, tightly wrapped in greaseproof paper, for an easy lunch.

Serves 4 (main meal) or 6 (light lunch)
4 eggs
450g/1lb/2–3C grated or chopped vegetables (carrot, parsnip, sweet potato, celery, etc.)
1 onion, chopped as finely as possible
1 green or red pepper (capsicum), chopped
115g/4oz/1C nuts, ground (walnuts, almonds, cashews, etc., but not peanut)
115g/4oz/1C cooked brown rice (about 85g/3oz/½C uncooked measure)
1 small sprig of fresh oregano or marjoram
salt and freshly ground black pepper

Method
Beat the eggs and combine with all the other ingredients. Place in a well-oiled baking dish and bake in a preheated oven at 190°C/375°F/gas mark 5 for 30 minutes or until cooked.

STIR-FRIED RICE AND BEANS

This can be a casual meal on its own, or it can be served with a side salad, or to accompany a meat or vegetable dish. The rice and beans can be either freshly cooked or can have been cooked and frozen. If they have been frozen, heat them through in boiling water before using. Alternatively you can add them frozen, and let them thaw out and heat up in the vegetables.

30ml/1½tbsp/2tbsp olive oil
4 fresh basil leaves (or other fresh herbs as available)
½tsp/1tsp ground coriander
¼tsp/½tsp ground cumin
a pinch of chilli powder (optional)
3 large cloves garlic, sliced
1 large onion, chopped
1 medium carrot, grated
4 peppers (capsicums), green, red, orange and yellow (if available), chopped
2 sticks celery, chopped
115g/4oz/1C cooked brown rice (about 85g/3oz/½C uncooked measure)
170g/6oz/1C cooked red kidney beans
salt and freshly ground black pepper

Method
Heat the oil in a frying pan or wok, add the fresh herbs and spices, and stir. Add the garlic and onion and sauté for a few minutes. Add the carrot, peppers and celery. When the vegetables are cooked add the rice and beans, stir, season and serve.

PASTA DISHES

When most people think of pasta dishes they think of rich tomato sauce. Since this usually involves tinned tomatoes, tomato purée or both, neither of which are permitted for you, I have included the following suggestions for home-made tomato sauces. Serve with spaghetti or other pasta dishes, either on their own or combined with your usual meat sauces.

TOMATO AND FENNEL SAUCE

Serves 2
1 medium onion, chopped
2 cloves garlic, chopped
30ml/1½tbsp/2tbsp olive oil
250g/8oz ripe tomatoes
1 red pepper (capsicum), chopped
1 green pepper (capsicum), chopped
salt and freshly ground black pepper
1–2tsp fennel weed

Method

Sauté the onion and garlic in the olive oil until the onion is transparent, then add the tomatoes and peppers. Season, add the fennel weed and continue to cook for 20 minutes. Add a cup of water and simmer for 1 hour, adding more water if necessary.

Serve over pasta, and sprinkle pine kernels over the top.

HOT TOMATO SAUCE

Serves 2
50ml/3tbsp/¼C olive oil
5 leaves fresh basil, chopped
250g/8oz tomatoes, chopped
2 cloves garlic, finely chopped
1 dried red chilli pepper (hot), deseeded and chopped
a pinch of cumin seeds
juice of 1 lemon
salt and freshly ground black pepper

Method

Heat the oil and sauté the garlic until golden then add the chilli, basil, cumin, and tomatoes, and season. Add the lemon juice and simmer for 1 hour.

Serve over freshly cooked pasta.

VEGETABLE DISHES

You may find that meals are less tasty when you eliminate the yeast-based foods from your diet. You may miss the various forbidden sauces – soya sauce, chilli sauce, tomato sauce and others. For this reason it's important to add interest with the vegetable dishes. This can be done with home-made sauces and fresh herbs. If you would normally add a dash of wine to a sauce, use brandy or whisky instead – but just a dash. Some suggestions are given below and these will also open your mind to other possibilities. The amount of flavourings, such as lemon juice, fresh herbs, etc., is up to you – so taste as you go along! In general, be generous with the herbs as they can help you to ring the taste changes and add variety to the meal.

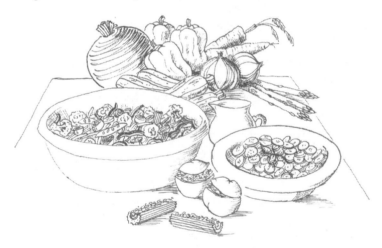

STUFFED VEGETABLES

You can stuff a great variety of vegetables, starting with the list below. Use garlic, spices and herbs such as basil, dill, oregano, marjoram, sage, thyme and fennel tops, and give the stuffing body with cooked brown rice and nuts. Cook extra rice in case you need it; you can always freeze it and use later. The vegetable shells can either be blanched (if you like them soft to eat) or used as they are (if you enjoy them slightly firm). Serve with a green salad.

Vegetables to stuff:

Capsicums or peppers   cut off the end with the stalk and remove and discard the centre and the seeds but chop any of the outside flesh you remove and set aside

Courgettes or zucchini and cucumbers   cut in half lengthways, scoop out the centre and set aside

Marrows or summer squash, butternut pumpkin and baby squash   cut in half lengthways, remove and discard the seeds (although some people like to include them, it is up to you), remove all the centre flesh, mash or grate it, depending on its consistency, and set aside

Onions   boil until softened, make a single cut from top to bottom and down one side only. Peel each outer layer off until you have several hollow onion balls, remove the inner, smaller layers, chop and set aside

Tomatoes   cut off the tops, hollow out the centre and set the pulp aside

Eggplants or aubergines   cut lengthways, remove all the centre flesh, chop and set aside

Celery stalks   choose large ones and cut into lengths of about 10cm/4in

Leeks   choose large ones and cut into lengths of about 10cm/4in, using the part held together by the root section, remove most of the inner leaves, chop and set aside

FOR THE STUFFING

The overall amount will depend on the quantity and type of vegetables to stuff, but work to the following guidelines.

50ml/3tbsp/¼C olive oil – or more: be generous
1 large onion, chopped
3 cloves garlic, crushed
1 bay leaf
1tbsp/2tbsp fresh herbs, chopped
½tsp/1tsp ground coriander
¼tsp/½tsp ground cumin
75g/2½oz/½C nuts, freshly ground or pulverized
115g/4oz/1C cooked brown rice (about 85g/3oz/½C uncooked
 measure)

Method

Sauté the garlic and onion in the olive oil. Chop or grate the parts of the vegetables set aside while creating the 'shells' for stuffing, then add to the pan and cook until softened.

Add the ground nuts and brown rice and mix thoroughly. The mixture should be firm enough to hold together; if not, add more rice: if you were conservative with the olive oil, add more now, it will contribute to the flavour.

When you can mould the stuffing into shapes, use it to fill all the prepared vegetable shells. Arrange them in a lightly oiled casserole dish, wedging them together so they prop each other up. Any spare stuffing can be spooned in between them as a base. Cook in a preheated oven at between 180°C/350°F/gas mark 4 and 205°C/400°F/gas mark 6 (the firmer and thicker the flesh the hotter the oven) for 40 minutes to 1¼ hours (the hotter the oven the shorter the time), according to the variety and the density of the stuffing.

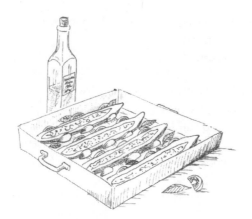

NUT-STUFFED CUCUMBERS

Serves 4

2 medium cucumbers
1 dried red chilli pepper (hot)
¼tsp/½tsp salt
1 large clove garlic, crushed
1 medium onion, chopped very fine
75g/2½oz/½C raw nuts, crushed
1tsp/2tsp poppy seeds
6 firm tomatoes, quartered
¼ lemon
8 fresh mint leaves
salt and freshly ground black pepper
20ml/1tbsp/1½tbsp olive oil
sunflower seeds to decorate

Method

Cut the cucumbers in half lengthways and scoop out the centre, leaving the skin on.

Chop and pulverize the chilli with the salt, then combine with the garlic and onion, and the crushed nuts and poppy seeds. Put this mixture into each of the 4 cucumber halves and arrange them in an oiled casserole dish with the tomatoes wedged around them for support. Squeeze the lemon juice over the tomatoes, cover with the mint leaves, drizzle the whole dish with the olive oil and bake, covered, in a preheated oven at 180°C/350°F/gas mark 4 for 1 hour. If it gets too dry, pour over a small amount of vegetable stock.

When it's cooked, sprinkle with sunflower seeds and place under the grill for 10 minutes.

Serve with brown rice and a side salad.

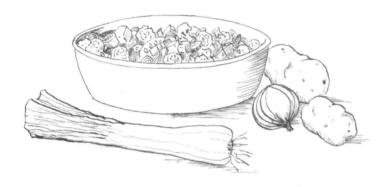

STEAMED MIXED VEGETABLES

This dish can be made with any variety of vegetables you have to hand and can be completed within fifteen minutes from start to serving. Cook your choice in this sequence: carrots, potatoes, parsnips, swedes or rutabagas, turnips, pumpkins and squashes, celery, onions, leeks, baby green beans, corn or sweetcorn, cauliflower and broccoli. Boil 2.5cm/1in of water in a pan with a tight-fitting lid. Using the vegetables you have chosen, or have to hand, and in the sequence given above, dice the root vegetables, one at a time and add to the boiling water, in sequence, as they are ready; similarly slice the celery, onion and leek, and add each one when it is ready, add the green beans and then the sweetcorn, finally break the cauliflower into small florets and add, then the broccoli. By the time you have added the last vegetables (the ones that need the least cooking) the root vegetables will be nearly cooked. You will just have time to lay the table before they are all ready. Serve with a meat or fish dish, with an omelette or with brown rice.

CARROTS WITH DILL

Serves 4
500g/1lb carrots
30g/1oz/2tbsp butter
1–2tbsp/2–4tbsp finely chopped fresh dill

Method
Slice the carrots and steam until tender. Toss in the butter, serve and sprinkle with dill weed. The exact amount will depend on your taste.

BAKED EGGPLANT OR AUBERGINE WITH PEPPERS

Serves 4
2 cloves garlic, thinly sliced
2 large onions, thinly sliced
2 eggplants or aubergines, sliced 1cm/½in thick (peel left on)
3 green and 3 red peppers (capsicums), thinly sliced
6 leeks, thinly sliced
6 basil leaves, chopped
50ml/3tbsp/¼C olive oil
juice of 1 lemon
salt and freshly ground black pepper

Method
Lightly oil a casserole dish and arrange the vegetables in alternating layers, sprinkling the last with the basil. Drizzle the olive oil over them, put the lid on the dish and bake in a preheated oven at

180°C/350°F/gas mark 4 for 2 hours; but for the last 15 minutes, squeeze over the lemon juice and cook with the lid off. Season and serve.

PIQUANT COURGETTES OR ZUCCHINI

Serves 2
60ml/3½tbsp/¼C/2tsp olive oil
1 clove garlic, chopped
6 spring onions
3 tomatoes, chopped
1 bay leaf
¼tsp/½tsp ground coriander
⅛tsp/¼tsp ground cumin
¼tsp/½tsp paprika
450g/1lb courgettes (zucchini)
¼ lemon
salt and freshly ground black pepper

Method
Heat the oil and sauté the garlic until lightly coloured. Cut the spring onions into 3cm/1in lengths and cut lengthways to make thin strips, then add to the pan until wilted. Add the tomatoes, bay leaf and spices and cook, stirring constantly, for 5 minutes, then add the courgettes (zucchini) and cook until soft.

Add the lemon juice, season and serve with brown rice.

LEMON–NUT SAUCE FOR VEGETABLES

Since sour cream is forbidden and you may not want to use butter, here is a useful sauce you can make in advance, store in the refrigerator, and pour over cooked vegetables to add interest.

2 cloves garlic, crushed
1½tbsp/2tbsp nut butter (almond butter, cashew butter, hazel nut
    butter, or tahini)
1½tbsp/2tbsp freshly squeezed lemon juice
2tbsp/3tbsp olive oil

Method
Combine the first three ingredients, mixing thoroughly. Slowly
add the olive oil, as if you were making mayonnaise, making sure
the mixture remains smooth. Add more oil if you would like a
thinner dressing, less if you want it to be thick. Store in the
refrigerator in an air-tight container.

SALADS

Salads provide endless opportunities to exercise the imagination.
You can use any of the salads you will find in any other recipe
book, just remember to leave out the mushrooms and to make your
own dressing.

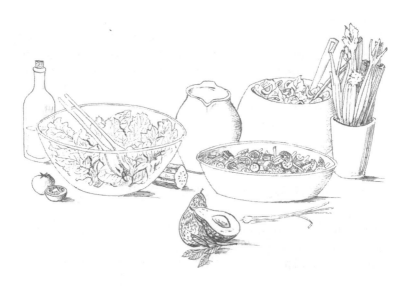

SALAD DRESSINGS

The major problem with salad dressing is the vinegar. As most commercial preparations are made with this, rather than lemon juice, it's important that you become comfortable with making your own dressings. The recipes below use lemon juice, but in all of them you can replace this with fresh grapefruit juice, orange juice or even apple juice (since the amount used is so small) unless your candida problem is severe.

LEMON MAYONNAISE

3 egg yolks
75ml/4tbsp/¹⁄₃C lemon juice
a pinch of English mustard powder (optional, to taste)
250ml/8fl oz/1C (approximately) olive oil
salt and freshly ground white pepper

Method
Put the egg yolks and lemon juice (and mustard powder if using) in a blender. Blend slowly. Keep the blender running and add the oil a few drops at a time. Continue adding the oil until you achieve the desired consistency. Adjust the seasoning towards the end, if necessary.

FRENCH DRESSING

3 parts olive oil
1 part freshly squeezed lemon juice
fresh herbs of your choice
garlic, finely chopped
salt and freshly ground black pepper to taste

Method
Combine all ingredients in a container with an air-tight lid and shake thoroughly. This will keep in the refrigerator for 1 week.

TAHINI DRESSING

tahini
water
freshly squeezed lemon juice
fresh herbs and/or crushed garlic
salt and freshly ground black pepper

Method
Put the required amount of tahini in a container, and add water slowly. Initially the mixture will thicken, then suddenly it will become very much thinner. Add sufficient lemon juice to balance the oil (a matter of taste) and sufficient water to provide the required degree of liquidity. Season.

COOKED SALAD DRESSING

250ml/8fl oz/1C milk
½tbsp/1tbsp wholemeal flour
2 eggs
75ml/4tbsp/⅓C olive oil
75ml/4tbsp/⅓C freshly squeezed lemon juice
English mustard powder (optional)
salt and freshly ground black pepper

Method
Combine the milk, flour, eggs and oil in a saucepan (a double boiler is helpful but not essential) and simmer until thick. Be careful not to allow the mixture to boil; keep below 90°C/200°F if possible. When thick, allow it to cool and beat in the mustard powder (if using) and lemon juice. Season and store in the refrigerator.

AVOCADO DRESSING

1 avocado
1 tomato
1tbsp/2tbsp chopped chives
up to 50ml/3tbsp/¼C olive oil
up to 50ml/3tbsp/¼C lemon juice
salt and freshly ground black pepper

Method
Place all the ingredients in a blender and blend until smooth. The amount of oil and lemon juice depend in part on the size of the avocado and in part on how thick or thin you want the dressing to be.

PARSNIPS WITH LEMON

Serves 2
250g/8oz parsnips
juice of 1 lemon

Method
Grate the parsnips, stir in the lemon juice and allow to stand for 1 hour.

PIQUANT AVOCADO SALAD

Serves 1
1 large avocado, peeled
   and stoned
1 white onion
3 medium celery stalks
100ml/4fl oz/½C
   lemon mayonnaise
½ lettuce

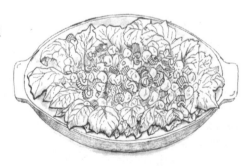

Method
Dice the avocado, chop the onion and celery, combine with lemon mayonnaise and serve on a bed of the lettuce.

TABBOULEH

Burghul is a type of cracked wheat; do not be tempted to use more; if you are wheat-sensitive you can use buckwheat (which is not a type of wheat).

Serves 4
2–3 *very* large bunches of oriental or flat-leafed parsley – this is the main ingredient of this dish
225g/8oz/1½C burghul
juice of 2 juicy lemons
4 large tomatoes, finely chopped
salt and freshly ground black pepper
a small bunch of spring onions, finely chopped (optional)
1 cos lettuce, leaves only

Method

Wash the parsley thoroughly, remove all stalks and chop finely.
   Soak the burghul in the lemon juice for 2 hours.
   Combine all the ingredients and serve immediately, using the lettuce leaves to scoop up the tabbouleh. Alternatively it can be eaten more conservatively, with a fork!

PEA AND PEPPER SALAD

Serves 2
1 avocado, diced
lemon mayonnaise (page 115)
salt and freshly ground black pepper
a small bunch of chives, chopped
450g/1lb (unshelled weight) peas, shelled and lightly cooked
1 orange and 1 yellow pepper (capsicum), diced
1 stick celery, diced
1 iceberg lettuce
3 tomatoes, quartered
a small handful of basil leaves, chopped

Method
Blend the avocado with lemon mayonnaise to taste, and season. Stir in the chives. Toss the peas, peppers and celery in this dressing and serve on a bed of lettuce leaves, surrounded by tomato wedges with the basil sprinkled over.

MANGETOUT AND POTATO SALAD

Mangetout peas are also known as snow peas, snap peas and sugar-snap peas. They do not need to be shelled, and are eaten whole.

Serves 2–4
200g/7oz mangetout
450g/1lb small new potatoes
1 yellow pepper (capsicum), chopped
2 spring onions, chopped
5 radishes, cut into rings
75ml/4tbsp/⅓C lemon mayonnaise (page 115)
75ml/4tbsp/⅓C French dressing (page 115)
1 lettuce
30g/1oz flaked almonds

Method
Boil the mangetout for 1 minute. Boil the potatoes until just cooked (be sure not to overcook them), and cut them into slices while still warm. Combine all the vegetables, then combine the two salad dressings and pour over the vegetables.

Toss lightly and serve in a salad bowl lined with lettuce leaves with the almonds sprinkled on top.

TOMATO AND BASIL SALAD

Serves 6
2 handfuls basil leaves, chopped
1kg/2¼lb tomatoes,
   sliced thinly
30ml/1½tbsp/2tbsp
   olive oil
1 lemon
salt and freshly ground
   black pepper

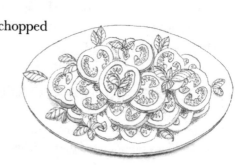

Method
Sprinkle the basil over the tomatoes, pour over the olive oil and mix gently. Squeeze sufficient lemon juice to give the desired piquancy. Season and serve.

DESSERTS

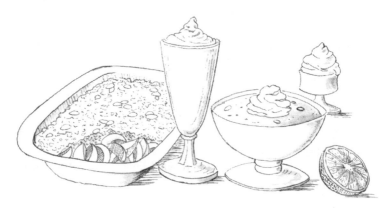

The majority of desserts are based heavily on white flour, sugar and cream and are not conducive to good health in anyone.

The usual healthy alternatives that are commonly suggested are either based on whole grains, fresh fruit and yoghurt or a variety of cheeses and biscuits. However, if you are suffering from candidiasis these are not workable solutions as yoghurt is not permitted, nor is cheese. In general, it is best to build the meal round savoury dishes and not to rely on a dessert course.

Creating 'permitted' desserts for people with candidiasis is a challenge, but it can be done. The aim in the recipes given below is to try to create the illusion of sweetness without adding sugar or honey. If your candida problem is mild you will be able to have a small amount of fruit, and for that reason some of the desserts do contain fruit. If your problem is very mild, even a very small amount of honey may be an 'acceptable cheat' occasionally. However, if you do have to avoid it, omit it from the recipes, they won't suffer.

CHILLED CARROT SPICE

Serves 2
170g/6oz/1C cooked and mashed carrots
75ml/4tbsp/⅓C single/light cream
nutmeg, cinnamon and cloves, to taste (or mixed spice)
1tsp/1tsp fresh lemon juice
1tsp/2tsp lemon zest
sesame seeds

Method
Place all the ingredients except the sesame seeds in a blender and blend until light and smooth. Pour into glasses and chill for 1 hour. Decorate with sesame seeds and serve.

COFFEE AND CAROB JELLY

Serves 2
500ml/16fl oz/2C strong black coffee
1tsp/2tsp powdered gelatine
3tbsp/6tbsp carob powder
a few drops vanilla essence, to taste
whipped cream

Method
Heat the coffee and dissolve the gelatine powder in it. Add the carob powder and vanilla essence and stir until smooth. Carob powder is slightly sweet and the vanilla will give an illusion of sweetness. Allow to cool and pour into a mould or into individual glasses when it is about to set.

Serve garnished with whipped cream.

CAROB AND PEPPERMINT JELLY

Serves 2
500ml/16fl oz/2C milk
1tbsp/2tbsp powdered
   gelatine
4tbsp/8tbsp carob powder
   (more or less to taste)
peppermint essence (to taste)
4 mint leaves

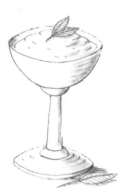

Method
Warm the milk, add the gelatine and stir until dissolved. Add the carob powder and peppermint essence. Stir until smooth, allow to cool and pour into glass dishes to set. Serve decorated with the mint leaves.

AVOCADO MOUSSE

Serves 2
2 avocados, peeled and stoned
2 eggs, separated
1 tbsp maple syrup (if permitted)
300ml/10fl oz/1¼C whipping/thick cream
50g/2oz chopped almonds

Method
Mash the avocados until smooth, then add the egg yolks (and the maple syrup if permitted) and beat until smooth. Whip the cream until stiff and fold it in, then whip the egg whites until stiff and fold them in. Spoon the mixture into dessert glasses and decorate with chopped almonds.

APPLE CRUMBLE

Serves 2–4
4 dessert apples, peeled, cored and sliced
170g/6oz/2C rolled oats or similar grain
1½tbsp/2tbsp tahini
50g/2oz flaked almonds
2tsp/2tsp liquid honey (this is a small cheat and should be omitted
   if you have to be strict)

Method
Simmer the apples in an absolute minimum of water, just sufficiently to soften them, then place them in a shallow baking dish. Combine the oats, tahini and honey (if used), then mix in half the almonds and spread this mixture over the apples. Sprinkle the rest of the flaked almonds over the top and bake in a preheated oven at 130°C/275°F/gas mark 1 for 40 minutes.

PEAR DUMPLINGS

Serves 4
½tsp/1tsp mixed spice
3tsp/6tsp lemon zest
1tbsp/2tbsp softened butter
4 large ripe pears, halved and cored
4 whole cloves
a little milk and butter
powdered cinnamon to decorate
Basic Pastry Variation (page 76), made with about 200g/7oz/
  1½C flour

Method
Combine the mixed spice, lemon zest and butter and place in the
hollows of the pears where the cores were. Place a clove nearer to
the top of one of the halves of each pear.

Roll about a quarter of the pastry as thinly as possible. Place the
two halves of one pear back together, lay the pear on the pastry and
fold the pastry over the top. Moisten the edges with milk, press
the pastry firmly together to make a sealed envelope and cut off the
excess pastry. The aim is to envelop the pear in a minimum amount
of pastry, so as to avoid a heavy dessert. Repeat with the other pears.

Place the dumplings in a buttered baking dish, brush them with
milk, dot them with butter and sprinkle with cinnamon. Bake in a
preheated oven at 180°C/350°F/gas mark 4 for 30 minutes.

Serve hot or cold, with Vanilla Cream (page 129).

STUFFED SWEET POTATOES

4 sweet potatoes
100ml/4fl oz/½C single/light cream
a pinch of freshly grated nutmeg
poppy seeds and fresh berries to decorate

Method
Wash the sweet potatoes and cut into serving sizes. Paint them

lightly with oil and bake in a moderate oven at 190°C/375°F/gas mark 5 for 45 minutes (or more or less depending on size).

Scoop out the centre of the potatoes, combine this with the cream and nutmeg and beat until smooth. Put the mixture back into the sweet potato shells and return to the oven until browned. Serve decorated with poppy seeds and berries.

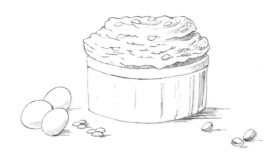

SWEET POTATO SOUFFLÉ

Serves 4
400g/14oz/2C mashed sweet potato (about 325g/11oz uncooked
   weight)
2 eggs, separated
1tsp/2tsp lemon zest
50ml/3tbsp/¼C double/heavy cream
50g/2oz/½C finely ground cashews or pine nuts
toasted flaked almonds to decorate

Method
Add the egg yolks, lemon zest and cream to the mashed sweet potatoes and beat thoroughly. Add the ground nuts. Whisk the egg whites until stiff (medium peak) and fold in. Bake in a preheated oven at 180°C/350°F/gas mark 4 for about 40 minutes, until light and slightly browned. Serve decorated with the toasted flaked almonds.

PUMPKIN PIE

Serves 4
Basic Pastry (pages 75–6) made with 115g/4oz/1C
2 C cooked and mashed pumpkin (butternut pumpkin is best)
2 eggs, separated
freshly grated nutmeg (to taste)
50ml/2fl oz/¼C whipping/heavy cream, whipped

Method
Line a 21cm/8in pie dish with the pastry.

Combine the pumpkin, egg yolks and nutmeg. Whip the egg whites until stiff and fold into the pumpkin mixture. Pile mixture into the pastry shell. Bake in a preheated oven at 180°C/350°F/ gas mark 4 for 45 minutes.

When cool decorate with the whipped cream and grated nutmeg.

CARROT PUDDING

Serves 4
200g/7oz/2C grated carrots
115g/4oz/1C finely ground nuts
50ml/2fl oz/¼C vegetable oil
140g/5oz/1C soya flour
zest of 1 orange
1tsp/2tsp nutmeg
1tsp/2tsp cinnamon
1tsp/2tsp cream of tartar

Method
Put the carrots, nuts and oil in a blender and blend thoroughly. In a bowl, combine the remaining ingredients, add the carrot mixture and stir thoroughly. Place in an oiled baking dish and cook in a preheated oven at 160°C/325°F/gas mark 3 for 3 hours.

Serve with a Nutty Milk (page 53).

RICE PUDDING

3–6 drops vanilla essence
brown rice, 50g/2oz/⅓C per person
milk
freshly grated nutmeg

Method
Add sufficient vanilla essence to the milk to make impart a strong flavour of vanilla. Add the brown rice to the milk and place in the top half of a double boiler. Place this over boiling water and allow to cook until the rice is soft. The amount of milk will depend on the type of brown rice, and how dry or moist you want the final result to be. Serve decorated with grated fresh nutmeg.

Variations
Use other spices, such as mace or cinnamon. Add grated rind of lemon or oranges. Add peppermint leaves to the milk and incorporate into the pudding; remove them before serving.

RICE FRITTERS

Rice Pudding made as in the previous recipe, but use *just* sufficient milk to cook the rice so that the final pudding is dry
1 egg for every 100g/3½oz/½C (raw) rice
butter for frying

Method
Beat the egg(s) and add to the rice pudding. Shape the mixture into balls, flatten, and fry lightly until golden.
   Serve with Vanilla Cream (page 129) or a Nutty Milk (page 53).

SPICED PANCAKES

Serves 2–4
8–12 Pancakes (page 60)
grated nutmeg
ground cinnamon
single/light cream

Method
Sprinkle the pancakes with grated nutmeg and powdered cinnamon, roll them up, and serve with cream.

Spiced Apple Pancakes
Serves 2–4
2 dessert apples, peeled, cored and sliced
8–12 Spiced Pancakes

Method
Steam the apples briefly until *just* tender and lay inside the pancakes before rolling them up.

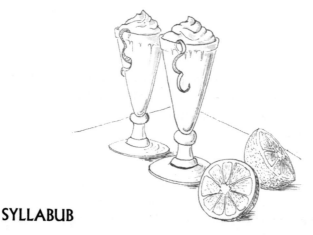

SYLLABUB

This may not be as sweet as the more common syllabub, but it is powerful! It is useful for dinner parties as it can be prepared in advance and kept in the refrigerator.

Serves 4
150ml/5fl oz/²/₃C whipping/heavy cream
175ml/6fl oz/³/₄C milk
50ml/3tbsp/¼C freshly squeezed orange juice
1tbsp/1½tbsp brandy
2 egg whites

Method

Combine the cream, milk, orange juice and brandy and whip until frothy. (Be careful not to turn it into butter.) Whip the egg whites until stiff and fold them into the mixture.

Chill and serve in slender glasses, decorated with a twist of orange rind.

VANILLA CREAM

Makes about 400ml/²/₃pt/1³/₄C
25g/1oz cornflour
1 large egg, separated
500ml/16fl oz/2C milk
1 vanilla pod, cut into pieces

Method

Make a paste with the cornflour, the egg yolk and some of the milk.

Using a double boiler, bring the rest of the milk to the boil with the vanilla pod, then pour it into the cornflour mixture, stirring all the time. Put this back in the double boiler and continue to heat gently until it has thickened. Strain to remove the vanilla pod at the last minute. This cream can be used instead of fresh cream, with other desserts.

PLANNING A MEAL OUT

In a Restaurant

There are many reasons for eating in a restaurant, from the need for a quick snack when hunger strikes, to the desire for a full and festive business or social occasion.

You may simply want a quick meal. If this is likely, use the strategies outlined in Chapter 10, Snacks and Light Lunches.

If you do decide to pop into a handy restaurant, then choose with care. Avoid snack bars where sandwiches are a major part of the offering. Avoid a pizza restaurant as you really are likely to find that there is nothing you can eat. Hamburgers are also out – without the bun they hardly provide a satisfying meal. At restaurants specializing in baked potato dishes you will have to avoid the baked beans, prawns in mayonnaise, coleslaw and cheeses, but tuna or salmon with corn and other similarly acceptable options are likely to be on offer. It can be helpful if you choose a restaurant where you can get a simple grill (meat, chicken or fish) with vegetables. Avoid Chinese restaurants as so many of the dishes are outside your range of choices; many already contain soya sauce, black bean sauce, oyster sauce and others, as well as tofu, a variety of mushrooms or sweet (sugar) sauces. Indian restaurants can be fairly safe, so can Lebanese restaurants, but in Thai restaurants you will have the problem of coconut in many dishes. Most European-cuisine restaurants will usually have some dishes you can choose.

When you go to a restaurant for a social evening keep in mind the reasons you are doing so. You are not going there solely to eat, there are many other benefits to the occasion. You are going for a pleasant night out, you are going for the atmosphere, the chance to talk to the people you are with, you are going so you don't have to cook or wash up, you are going so you can relax. All these benefits will still apply, even if you can't eat the food of your choice. How much you enjoy the occasion will then depend, to a large extent, on your attitude and what you are saying to yourself, and to others. Ideally you would be wise to make no comment about the dishes you cannot have. Instead, make your choice from the ones you can have, select it and let the other people think it's your first choice. There will then be nothing to discuss and you can join in and enjoy the conversation without the cloud of discontent that could otherwise occur. If you are hungry, have a starter or order extra vegetables. There will be nothing on the dessert trolley or the cheese board that you can have, except possibly fresh fruit, which you can have if your problem is mild.

Dealing with a Fixed Menu

When the meal is set, and you have no choice, there can be a more difficult problem.

If you are going to a friend's home the best thing, usually, is to give them a list of the foods you cannot eat and some suggestions of what you can – even lend them this book! If you tell them what you can have, make sure that it will fit in with what they are serving and with a minimum of extra work for your hostess. Let them know that if they plan a meal you can eat you will be thrilled and very appreciative, but if, on the other hand, the meal they have planned to serve contains a variety of things you can't have you will be perfectly happy with, for instance, the vegetables, and a simple piece of grilled chicken. It's up to you to assure your hostess that you will be totally satisfied with the result – even if you are secretly drooling over the delicious, but forbidden, meal she has prepared for everyone else. Another alternative is to offer to bring for yourself a meal that you can eat. If you want to be inconspicuous, make it, at least superficially, as similar to theirs as you can. Which option you choose will depend on how well you know your hostess, the other people involved and the various foods on offer.

If you are going to a formal dinner or one catered for by caterers or a hotel, for instance, the problem and hence the solution will be different. You may be able to explain the situation to the organizers and ask them to prepare a special meal. If so, give them a list of the foods you cannot have and ask them to make sure they are all excluded. If this is not possible, or if you feel uncomfortable doing this, there are still ways around it. One is to make sure you have something to eat before you go; not a lot, but sufficient to kill the hunger pangs. In this situation, if there are parts of the meal you cannot eat you can simply leave them, and eat what you can. Even if there is only a small amount you can eat, you won't be excessively hungry at the end. Another alternative is to carry the ubiquitous bag of nuts (not peanuts) with you. Eat what you can of the meal and fill up on nuts. You could, of course, take some other snack food with you, but nuts are compact, long-lasting, need no preparation and are very filling.

Remember in all these situations: the food is not the only issue. There is the whole occasion to enjoy. Keep in mind too that you're not purely suffering deprivation. You are also making great strides back to health.

CHAPTER 13

Drinks

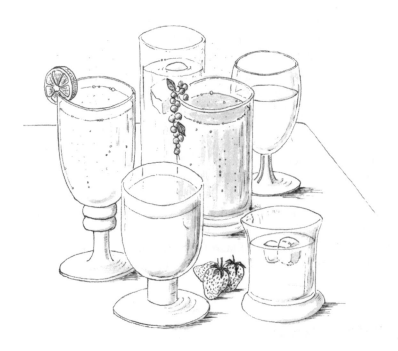

Not only is there a list of foods that you must avoid on a candidiasis treatment diet, there is also a list of drinks. In fact knowing what you can and can't drink is just as important as knowing what you can and can't eat.

HOT DRINKS

Many of the normal hot drinks are available to you, provided you don't add sugar. Coffee may not be good for you, or for anyone, but it probably won't worsen the candida problem in the way high-yeast or sugar-based foods can. You may also be able to drink tea successfully. However, if your candidiasis is severe the small amounts of mould that can collect on tea leaves may aggravate the problem, in which case you should avoid it.

Cereal coffees, otherwise known as coffee substitutes, can also be drunk. Dandelion coffee, made from the dried ground root, is not only pleasant in flavour – it's my favourite hot drink – but good for the liver and kidneys, organs that are under stress in candidiasis. Most instant versions of dandelion coffee contain the milk sugar lactose. If your problem is mild this may not matter. If it is severe you should avoid the lactose: purchase the pure dried and ground dandelion root, pour boiling water on it, allow it to simmer for ten to twenty minutes and then strain before serving. You can have milk with any of these drinks, provided you are not allergic or sensitive to it, but not sugar.

Herb teas can contain moulds. If your problem is mild, the amount you get from an occasional cup of herb tea may not matter; however, where possible make the tea from the fresh leaves. If your problem is severe it is essential that you use fresh rather than dried leaves.

COOL DRINKS

Fruit juices and soft drinks are *out*, they contain too much sugar and will almost certainly encourage the growth of *Candida albicans*.

If you absolutely must have a sweet drink you could use some of the artificially sweetened drinks without risking your treatment, but there is then the risk of the problems caused by the sweeteners, the possibility of liver problems or cancer, from aspartame, cyclamates and saccharine. The risks are small – you may consider them acceptable – but they are there none the less.

Keep heart, though, there are a variety of possibilities, in addition to pure water, such as those listed below. Not only do they taste pleasant, they can and should be made to look appealing. You are already going without a great deal: attractive presentation can lift your spirits.

As well as providing pleasant flavours, some of these drinks will not only avoid doing you harm but can also help you overcome some of your symptoms. See the use of sage and thyme for sore throats and a variety of seeds for the gas, wind and bloating.

COOL MINERAL WATERS

The quantities are for one glass; if you want more, scale them up accordingly.

Lemon Mineral Water
still mineral water
2 slices of lemon
ice cubes

The lemon is sufficient to provide a refreshing flavour without creating too much bitterness.

Pink Fizz
aerated mineral water
a few drops of Angostura bitters
1 strawberry
ice cubes

Make a cut halfway through the strawberry and wedge this on the rim of the glass, to decorate; and yes, you can eat it afterwards.

Cranberry Soda
¾ glass aerated mineral water
¼ glass cranberry juice

Natural cranberry juice, like lemon juice, contains a negligible amount of sugar. Be sure that you do not buy one to which sugar or other fruit juices have been added. Cranberry juice has the added advantage of being beneficial to the kidneys and urinary tract and so can help some of the problems caused by the candida.

COOL TEAS

In the sense used here a 'tea' is an infusion made by pouring boiling water onto the flavouring substance, which is usually the leaves of the herb, and sometimes the seeds.

Any herb teas that you enjoy hot can also be drunk cold. However they should, where possible, be made from fresh herbs rather than from dried herbs since dried herbs can carry moulds. If you cannot readily buy the fresh herbs that you like buy the plants. They can be grown in the garden, in tubs on balconies and patios, and even indoors as pot plants.

Try the lemon flavours such as lemon balm and lemon grass. Peppermint and camomile are popular. As you grow bold experiment with others.

A common problem if candida in the digestive tract moves up above the stomach and into the throat and mouth, is frequent sore throats. Sage and thyme can help. Add boiling water to the leaves and allow them to infuse. The teas can be drunk hot or cold and will help relieve both a sore throat (especially when it and/or your tongue has a white coating) and the flatulence and bloating.

For best results allow the infusion to cool and then gargle with it. Drinking the infusion regularly will help to keep the problem at bay.

COOL SPICE DRINKS

The traditional drink for most Europeans to have with a curry is beer. This is definitely to be avoided if you have candidiasis. However you can do yourself a double favour with spices since they both taste nice and improve your digestion.

In many countries seeds such as those of caraway, cumin, cardamom, fennel, aniseed, dill and pimento (often known as 'allspice' and not to be confused with 'mixed spice', made from cinnamon, cloves and nutmeg) are placed on the table after a meal in small dishes for people to nibble. They are pleasant in flavour and help to reduce dyspepsia and flatulence, two problems you are probably experiencing.

To make a pleasing cool drink, pour boiling water on the seeds you have chosen and then allow to infuse until cold. Strain before serving. If you like more flavour you could simmer the seeds in boiling water for ten to fifteen minutes before allowing to cool. Serve with a mint leaf as decoration, or even for flavour. This also aids digestion.

ALCOHOLIC DRINKS

There are going to be problems for you associated with drinking alcohol, since the majority of alcoholic drinks contain yeast, sugar or both.

From the avoidance list at the beginning of the dietary section you will recall that you must avoid – totally – beer, wine, champagne, sherry, port, vermouth and all similar drinks. All liqueurs must be avoided because of their sugar content. The only alcohol you can have is in the form of non-sweet neat spirits such as whiskey, gin, brandy or vodka – not rum, for instance, as it is too sweet. If your problem is severe you may find that even these cause aggravation of your symptoms, but many people can drink them successfully.

The next step is to consider what you can drink with them, since so many of the 'splits' contain sugar. Keep in mind that the aim here is twofold. Firstly you want a drink you can enjoy. You may not enjoy some of the following suggestions *as much as* your favourite wine or beer, but do pick the best of the bunch. Secondly, you want to be seen to be drinking socially with your friends and not being a party pooper. So even if these drinks do not come high on your favourite drink list, make a good show of it, pretend you are enjoying them and that they are your real choice for the moment. That way you will at least avoid the ribbing that goes with people trying to persuade you that 'just a little wine won't matter', when you know perfectly well that it will.

WHISKEY / WHISKY

You have it easy. You can drink it neat or add water, soda water or ice, just as you normally do.

GIN AND VODKA

These can be drunk just like whisky/whiskey. Artificially sweetened tonics are sugar-free.

Martini and Vodka Martini
Gin and vodka drinkers can still have their martini so long as they like it so dry they won't miss even the single drop of vermouth. In other words it will actually be neat gin, served, if you like, with ice and a slice of lemon. Remember that you can no longer have the olive as this may be carrying yeasts.

Pink Gin
A Pink Gin, with 1–2 drops of Angostura bitters, is also acceptable, with or without mineral water to make it a long drink. Again you can also use vodka in the same way.

Sloe Gin

Sloes can be bitter and are normally added to the gin in combination with sugar. As you know you cannot add sugar, so it is time to be creative. Consider adding a variety of other fruits to the gin instead. You are adding them mainly for the flavour so base your choice on that. For gooseberry gin, fill a bottle up to the neck with gooseberries, pour in sufficient gin to fill in all the spaces and cover even the topmost gooseberry, allow to stand for six months – or as long as your self-restraint lasts – and drink neat or with ice, soda or mineral water. Alternatively, copy the Gooseberry Gin recipe but use raspberries instead. If you would like to strengthen the colour add a few drops of beetroot juice (you won't taste it, but you will certainly see the colour). Serve with soda and ice, and decorate with a mint leaf and a slice of orange.

Brandy, Cognac and Armagnac

These are all safe to drink as they are commonly drunk neat. Brandy and soda is also a safe drink. These drinks can all be drunk whenever you want a drink, such as before dinner, in the pub or at a bar. They can also be drunk with meals, American style, instead of wine.

ALCOHOL ALTERNATIVES

If you are not a heavy drinker and not a wine buff – in other words, you only drink socially, when the occasion demands it – the problem may not be what to drink now that some of your favourites are denied to you, but how to look socially acceptable and avoid unwanted comments. In other words, what do you do when you are out socially, everyone else is drinking and you don't want to make a fuss or look out of things? Here are some practical suggestions.

Mineral 'Wine'

Ask for a wineglass and drink the mineral water from that. Simply using the same shaped glass as the others at the table means most people quickly forget you are not drinking wine like everyone else, and you blend in.

L'Eau Rosé

Adding a drop of Angostura bitters to the mineral water will impart a colour that mimics a rosé wine.

Innovative 'Red Wine'

One client went a step further. She did enjoy alcohol and friends knew she normally drank red wine. On social occasions she carried with her a small flask of gin with some beetroot juice (available from health-food shops) as colouring. A small amount of this, added to the mineral water in her wineglass, looked like red wine, tasted, as she said, a bit like a diluted martini and was an acceptable substitute until she became healthy again.

'Gin and Tonic'

If you are drinking at a party or in the pub and don't want to be a party pooper, yet don't like spirits, remember, a glass of mineral water with ice and a slice of lemon looks just like a gin and tonic. Just make sure you have the appropriate glass and sip rather than gulp. Some of my patients have even chosen to drink gin diluted with mineral water.

CHAMPAGNE?

For that very special occasion, when you're simply not going to stick to your boring old diet, avoid beer, avoid wine, insist on champagne – and make sure it is French, not one of the many champagne-style wines, excellent though many of them are, from other countries. The French ones seem to have the smallest amount of yeast left in. However this *is* breaking the diet so stick to one glass and only do it at weddings and (major!) anniversaries.

Conclusion

The treatment of *any* health problem from a naturopathic point of view includes considering and working with the whole person. This is *particularly* true and particularly necessary in the case of candidiasis.

The problem, by its very nature, is one that involves the whole person and all aspects of life. There is no point in looking for a pill to kill the bug. In the case of *Candida albicans*, you could never kill them all, and it only takes a few to rebuild the colony. This is why the medical solution, an anti-fungal medication, is not effective. Even if you kill off most of the yeast cells, the ones that remain are left in the same environment as encouraged their growth beforehand. So there is no point in treating the problem as if it was localized to the vagina, the digestive tract or even the fingernails or between the toes. The whole person is the environment in which the candida was able to do so well in the first place and it is the whole person that must be changed for the problem to be solved.

As you have discovered, eradicating the problems caused by an excessive growth and presence of *Candida albicans* involves even more than working holistically with the body. It involves what you eat and drink, it involves your clothes, your sexual activities, your habitat and how you maintain the environment around you. It involves your family and social life because your eating restrictions will have a bearing on what the people around you eat.

It also means working with the emotions, both those caused by the candida directly and those resulting from having to deal with the problem. It is certainly true that many emotional imbalances you may be experiencing come as a direct result of the chemical changes caused by the candida. However, while these will resolve once you have brought the candida under control, you may well benefit from emotional help and support while these changes are being brought about. You may also benefit from emotional help in relation to the frustrations you feel as a result of the restrictions that are being imposed.

Candida is a systemic problem in the fullest sense of the word. As such the natural therapies and some of the alternative forms of psychotherapy are far better suited to its treatment than is conventional medicine. What you have been given here can help you with your diet and ease your path to better health. You have also learnt about some of the supplements and remedies, the vitamins, minerals, herbs and homoeopathics, that can help you to beat the problem and rebuild your health.

If you want further help there are many naturopaths, many natural therapists, who can provide this. Look for one who specializes in the treatment of this problem and who uses a variety of different approaches. You want more than someone who is a dedicated homoeopath, or a dedicated herbalist or even a dedicated nutritionist. You want someone who combines all these therapies, and more, to help you with all the different aspects of the problem. They will then be able to tailor the treatment to your own specific needs and deal with any associated problems you may have.

This book is a start. It may of itself be sufficient to help you solve the problem, but be reassured: if it is not, there is more help out there – the problem can be beaten.

Useful Organizations and Further Reading

USEFUL ORGANIZATIONS

Australia and New Zealand

Australian Natural Therapists Association
PO Box 308
Melrose Park
South Australia 5039
Tel 8 8297 9533
Fax 8 8297 0003

Australian Traditional Medicine Society
PO Box 442 or Suite 3, First Floor
120 Blaxland Road
Ryde
NSW 2112
Tel 2 9808 2825
Fax 2 9809 7570

New Zealand Natural Health Practitioners Accreditation Board
PO Box 37–491
Auckland
Tel 9 625 9966

North America

American Association of Naturopathic Physicians
PO Box 20386
Seattle
WA 98102
Tel 206 323 7610
Fax 206 323 7612

American Holistic Medical Association
4101 Lake Boone Trail, Suite 201
Raleigh
NC 27607
Tel 919 787 5146
Fax 919 787 4916

Canadian Holistic Medical Association
700 Bay Street
PO Box 101, Suite 604
Toronto
Ontario M5G 1Z6
Tel 416 599 0447

Diagnos-Tech
620 South 192nd
#J-104
Kent
WA 98032
(1-800-87-TESTS)
For information about testing.

Great Smokies Diagnostic Laboratory
18a Regent Park Blvd
Asheville
NC 28806
Tel 1 800 522 4762
For information about testing.

International Health Foundation
PO Box 3494
Jackson
TN 38303
Tel 901 427 8100
Fax 901 423 5402
The Foundation will provide a list of doctors in the USA and Canada who are interested in yeast-related illness.

Dr Robert F Cathcart MD
127 Second Street
Los Atlos
California 94022
Tel 415 949 2822

Southern Africa

South African Homeopaths, Chiropractors and Allied Professions Board
PO Box 17055
0027 Groenkloof
S Africa
Tel 2712 466 455

United Kingdom

Action for ME
PO Box 1302
Wells BA5 1YE
Tel 01749 677 551
Web site: http://www.afme.org.uk

British Association for Counselling
37a Sheep Street
Rugby
Warks CV21 3BY
Tel 01788 578328

British Association of Nutritional Therapists
PO Box 47
Heathfield
East Sussex TN21 8ZX

British Holistic Medical Association
179 Gloucester Place
London NW1 6DX
Tel 0171 262 5299

Candida Support Network

Gibliston Mill
Colinsburgh
Leven
Fife
Scotland KY9 1JS
Tel 0133 340311

A UK database has been set up to put fellow sufferers living near each other in touch, in order for them to meet up informally or to set up a support group. Details of up and running groups are also given. Send £5 and a sae to the above address.

Candida Web Site

http://ourworld.compuserve.com/homepages/candida

For workshop details, support group contacts, details of books and tapes, treatments and research.

Council for Complementary and Alternative Medicine

179 Gloucester Place
London NW1 6DX
Tel 0171 724 9103
Fax 0171 724 5330

Diagnos-Tech

The Cottage
Lakeside
180 Lifford Lane
Kings Norton B30 3NT
Tel 0121 458 3407
Fax 0121 459 1656

For testing: Yeast Screen-CandaScan, CS1 Stool Culture for Yeast and Mucosal Barrier Screen.

General Council and Register of Naturopaths

2 Goswell Road
Street
Somerset BA16 0JG
Tel 01458 840072

Institute for Complementary Medicine and British Register of Complementary Practitioners
PO Box 194
London SE16 1QZ
Tel 0171 237 5165
Fax 0171 237 5175

National Candida Society
PO Box 151
Orpington
Kent BR5 1UJ
Membership £15 pa.

National Institute of Medical Herbalists
56 Longbrook Street
Exeter
Devon EX4 6AH
Tel 01392 426022
Fax 01392 498963

Register of Nutritional Therapists Ltd
Hatton Green
Warwick CV35 7LA

USEFUL FURTHER READING

Crook, William G, *The Yeast Connection*, Dakota, 1986.
Orion Truss, C, *The Missing Diagnosis*, Alabamah, 1983.

Index